CW01522256

HEAVY YEARS

ALSO BY AUGUSTUS YOUNG

AUTOFICTION

Light Years

Storytime

The Nicotine Cat and other people

Brazilian Tequila

POETRY

On Loaning Hill

The Credit

Lampion and His Bandits: Literature of the Cordel in Brazil

Days and Nights in Hendon

M.emoire

PLAYS

The Invalidity of All Guarantees

HEAVY YEARS

Inside the Head of a
Health Worker

Augustus Young

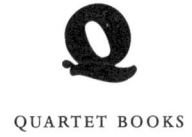

QUARTET BOOKS

First published in 2018 by Quartet Books Limited
A member of the Namara Group
27 Goodge Street, London, W1T 2LD

A catalogue record for this book is available from the British Library

ISBN 9780704374478

Typeset by Tetragon, London
Printed and bound in Great Britain by TJ International Ltd, Padstow, Cornwall

Although based on real events, some names have
been changed to maintain confidentiality

'The author has the right to use what he himself has experienced. But he must keep the truth to himself and only let it be refracted in various ways.'

—'The Law of Delicacy'
Søren Kierkegaard

'Medicine is a social science, and politics is nothing but medicine on a larger scale.'

—Rudolf Virchow

CONTENTS

PROLOGUE

Who is Talking
in My Head?

'Then seek no more out of thyself to find
The thing that thou hast sought so long before,
For thou shalt find it sitting in thy mind.'

—'Satires'
Thomas Wyatt

THE STRANGE BOY

M Y EARLY LIFE WAS A MAGIC LANTERN SHOW. THE hand rabbits were brothers and sisters, shadowy creatures who appeared to be in competition with me. I wondered what game we were playing, and what the house rules were. It all seemed rather makeshift, subject to outside forces. A big person came into the room, turned off the light, and told me to go to sleep. But I didn't like my dreams. Sometimes I woke up in the middle of the night and wanted to scream. I was afraid for myself in the dark, but in dreams I was afraid of myself.

The walls of the nursery were brownish yellow with damp. I waited for the life outside myself to begin again. The light, filtering through narrow latticed windows, more often than not, oozed grey from drizzle. Eventually someone would come to permit me to get up.

My life as a puppet didn't last. I outgrew my cot, and my pram was taken over by a bundle of swaddling clothes. I was expected to stand on my own two feet. I tottered into the arms of a woman, not my mother. I didn't like her any more than my dreams. She was all elbows, but broke my fall. I was put back on my feet. I was no longer afraid, and deliberately walked in puddles, and ate earth. When the time to be washed came, my mother complained, but I wasn't blamed. A word was had with the Polish student who looked after me. There was a war on.

I felt that I was getting away with something all the time. I didn't know what. It wasn't my attraction to dirt. That was obviously spotted. I moved on to eating nettles. By bypassing the lips to grind with the teeth I could avoid being stung. But it wasn't that I was getting away with. My parents were none the wiser. When my father saw me coming home with a green face and covered in mud, he said, 'that boy hasn't a thought in his head. All he does is run around. Clearly there is something wrong.' Or right, my mother hoped. I had been a difficult birth, coming early and upside down. A knife was necessary.

I grasped that nobody knows what you're thinking. Far from being a thoughtless boy, I was thinking all the time. Mostly of how not to upset the kindly people who troubled themselves with me. Needlessly, I thought. I was perfectly happy to be left alone. I would have liked to be the outsider looking in, unbeknownst. But I was trapped on the inside looking out, and up. And when I escaped and did what I wanted, it could be a problem, sometimes for me.

That my three siblings were more at home was evidenced by their puzzled looks when I came into the room. It crossed my mind that I could be a changeling, like the one in the poem my father recited: 'Come away, O human child/ to the waters and the wild/ with a faery, hand in hand,/ for the world's more full of weeping than you can understand.' The more familiar I became with their goings-on the stranger I felt. The siblings laughed a lot and I thought it must be their way of hiding the weeping. The baby, Michael, who took over my pram, fitted in as though to the manner born. If I knew about hospitals I would have asked my mother if there could have been a mix up.

I soon realised that the rules of the game of growing up were opportunist. For instance, the first choice of sweet cakes from town for Sunday tea was granted by relative age and size.

But grace and favour also played its part. If you were cute like Michael you could leapfrog to a poppy seed cake. Make yourself useful to older sisters by running messages, and the world's your chocolate eclair. I didn't play the game out of cussedness, and usually ended up with the last cake. But even if I revolted by breaking the plate, nothing too dreadful would happen. Threats of reformatory school, or being sold to the tinkers, were idle. Parents didn't throw children out.

I accepted my lot, aware that good losers had something to gain. When my younger brother, who called himself Eglantine, learned to read before me, he celebrated by jumping around, and proclaiming me the fool of the family. Infant fierceness made me want to throw myself on the ground, and kick my legs in the air. I restrained myself, and my father, who was teaching us, knocked the smirk off Eglantine's face with a look. A precocious paragon had higher expectations to live up to. I wore my dunce's cap with impunity.

COURT OF APPEAL

The benevolence of parents had a larger dimension. It came with duty, often painful, and what they called 'your own good'. Praise was measured for high achievers, and the prospect of retribution more to the fore. My mother led in everyday matters of crime and punishment, and dispatched her role impatiently, without satisfaction. I sympathised with her, not doubting that I, for one, was owed the ritual slap with the flat of a wooden spoon on the palm of the hand, even when found wanting for the wrong reason. Sins of thought are inviolable secrets.

My father was kept in reserve for questions of faith and morals. His judgements were absolute and clear. He held court with judicious aplomb, regulated by reasonableness, and avoidance of doubt. When in the dock I found it difficult to sit still. And couldn't help smiling to myself. How could I be the cause of such weighty deliberations? But his even-handedness prolonged the discourse. I couldn't wait for the rebuke to be delivered. It tended to come with a pat on my bowed head, as though approving me as a sounding board for larger moral concerns.

My mother's chastisements upset me most when she went beyond a quick slap. Eglantine would come running to her after I roughed him up in a jealous rage, and she prophesied, 'Your temper will see you hanged yet,' and promised to beat me 'to within an inch of your life,' which meant merely a look of quiet despair at what she had brought into the world.

Somehow my crimes and our mutual punishment did not seem commensurate. I deliberately misbehaved in order to make the perceived errors of my ways justify an indulgence of impulse. For instance, a healthy wallop when I put rotten apples in Eglantine's bed left no hard feelings. On the other hand, the predicted hanging lingered, and I came to anticipate it as a moment of closeness between us. I, the eldest son, the felon, lifted to the scaffold, while she quietly felt the shame of it. My speech from the dock would be semi-noble. 'Punish me, but not my mother. She deserved better. Still, Eglantine was asking for it.'

I could even claim my bad behaviour distracted my mother from more serious concerns. She might be the hand behind the magic lantern show, but my father's sleep was the presiding household god, always invoked in hushed tones. He worked at night on his books and papers, and slept by day. When the door of his bedroom opened like the heavens, and a wounded voice would say, 'I'm attempting to sleep. Please *try* and control those children of *yours*,' my mother was not best pleased. 'Trying' was an expression not tolerated by my mother. You *did*, or you *didn't*. The consequent punishment included my mother punishing herself. We were her fault.

My persecution of Eglantine was not unwelcome amongst my siblings. His blue-and-white knitted suits and curly black hair made him a street darling, but he was a holy terror in the house. For instance, he learned to spit on the Sunday cake of his choice as a sure way of getting it. And so I was merely enacting what they wanted to do themselves. But any suspicion that I might be acting on their behalf needed to be allayed or they would turn on me. And so I let it be known I was doing it because he was *their* pet.

Being seen to do the wrong thing for the right reason (or was it the other way round?) gave me pause. I wasn't getting away with it any more. People were seeing me in my own mirror. Fired by the thought that Eglantine's success with older women in the village was at my expense, I had set myself up to get caught with the apple-bed. If only, I thought ruefully, the family and I could agree again that I was just a silly boy without a thought in the world, everything would be all right.

I played fond and foolish as the defender of my little brother with the rough boys down the road. But Eglantine said 'only a fool or you' (a surprise compliment that has served me well throughout my life). He had moved on. The cute little outfits and curls disappeared into a crew cut, and tight-fitting corduroys, and he reverted to being called Michael. He could look after himself.

I was sent to the nuns' school, where I was the only boy. It was felt that a missionary order would know how to deal with my untamed impulses. But the nuns took my aberrant behaviour seriously, having recently come to believe that savages were best converted by allowing them to be more themselves. That was how to find 'the real person and nurture his innate goodness'. When the nuns encouraged me to be 'more myself' I was confused. I regarded myself as the mock-up of a real person, and my life as something of a dummy run.

THE WRITING ON THE WALL

At key points of my life the cinema has served me like Belshazzar's writing on the wall. This magic lantern show was more real to me than its nursery precursor. It took place in a palace, in colours more vivid than life. The screen was flat, but as it absorbed me, I was on the outside looking into a three-dimensional world. However, unlike the last king of Babylon, the writing on the wall didn't predict my downfall. This light shining in my darkness was a forewarning to accommodate my little self to the larger realities outside it.

I asked my mother what the coded message written by a disembodied hand on the wall of the king's banquet meant, and she improvised:

MENE: I have what you need.
TEKEL: You take more than is necessary.
UPHARSIN: Give back the surplus and let's split the difference.

This interpretation became mine while watching *Lili*. In the film a crippled soldier expresses his feelings for an orphan girl, Lili, through the strings he pulls as a fairground puppeteer. It ends in friendship, which means she pushes his wheelchair sometimes. As I left the cinema, I knew my mother was right, and what you get with love is the split difference between what's on offer and what you need. I learned to keep my feelings on a string, and bide my time until I was found out.

The cinema was where I shed the chrysalis of childhood. I realised there was a world outside me that wasn't merely rules to be got around. The butterfly of ambiguity fluttered in the air, and alighted on me, banishing the boring certitudes of everyday life. Touched by the light and sound of this other world, the mind was cleared of preconceptions, and I felt anything was possible. Before the main feature, Fred Bridgeman, the organist, rising up from the pit on his golden chariot, was God. The screen threw a coat of many colours on the audience, the tattoo of Hollywood, a seance that spirited up not the dead past but the future to be lived. In the end when the lights came back up, the butterfly flew off, but life had been given a metaphorical release that added a new dimension to my world.

DEAD BAT

An attempt to settle me in a boarding school failed. I ran away during the second term. The mark it left on me was a sleep complex. Fearing what the other boys might get up to, I slept as lightly as possible, with a crystal set tuned to pirate radio, and a hand torch under the covers. Giant shadows loomed above me. I finished the year in the local National school. Most of the village children would leave school at fourteen and go into apprenticeships or service. Beatings were routine. A switch of hazel to the back of the legs whipped the boys and girls into shape. There were two teachers. Mrs Hobson who had a nose like the knob of a blackthorn stick. And Skin the Goat, who had been a student of my father and venerated him. I was spared the rod by not being posed questions in class (I could ask them). And privileged to make the fire each day, a task I loved. I came to school early and collected dry wood in the undergrowth of the grounds. I was never happier than watching the kindling dancing into flame, and putting logs on to heat the pipes which were lined with bottles of milk for the pupils' lunch.

When exams came around Mrs Hobson used me as an invigilator, and I assisted her in collating the papers. I was allowed to mark myself. When the results were sent home my mother said, 'There must be some mistake, or the boy is a genius.' I immediately confessed all. She didn't tell my father.

During the long summer holidays a cricket pitch was carved out of some wasteland. The boys picked up the rules from listening to the BBC. We played for hours with a stone ball and a planed baseball bat. I was called the hindrance, being nearly impossible to bowl out. I covered the stumps with a dead bat, playing no strokes. Any runs I made were off the edge. Thirteen not out was my highest score. Nought not out meant I was on form.

That autumn I was sent to the Christian Brothers to toughen me up. Accustomed to small classes, I was so overwhelmed by the sheer numbers and noise that I can only describe the experience in terms of the expressionist film *Metropolis*. The school, built on a steep slope, resembled an air-raid shelter under a sheer cliff. Hundreds of boys hung on by invisible cables controlled by an unseen power. As they struggled in the air, some of them pulled at one another, and fell off from time to time. The mass of boys clung together in a choir, alternating between plainchant (for the teachers) and rugby songs (for themselves).

In this hanging prison, punishment was random. All you could do was to hope for the best of the worst. The notion of courting better risked strangulation. I was no trapeze artist and often lost my footing, clinging on by a bootstrap. I showed some ability in tying myself up in knots, but that twisted the cables, and their holders cut me loose. I was in free fall. Still the system was elastic, and at the last moment before hitting the ground I ricocheted back in the harness. As with my infancy in the family, there was always a release clause from the worst of the worst.

I had moved from an uncertain world to a preordained one, and took stock. I knew about original sin, but I was damned if my place in the world could be predetermined by a burden everybody was said to share. Not that the other boys seemed to suffer. They fought their corner, behind the backs of the Brothers. Dirtily for the most part. 'Survival is the name of the game,' was often said, while keeping to the letter rather than to the spirit of the law. I didn't want to abide by either, but remained passive, biding my time. 'Courage,' I said. 'I will swing into place once I catch up with myself.' The others were not going to drag me down.

I found the best way of resisting the pull was not by duplicitous conformity, but by creating a strain between me and the Brothers. My experience as a hindrance at cricket stood me in good stead. I said as little as possible in class, stonewalling questions with a humbly whispered 'I don't know'. Asked to participate in extra-curricular activities, such as the school play or choir, I said I'd prefer not to. I could have excused myself with lies, or offered myself to the school orchestra. My parents had signed me on for violin lessons in town, thinking if all else failed I'd get a busker spot outside Woolworths. I had a penchant for double-stopping. Playing two strings at the same time.

My dead-bat stance went down well with the boys. Remembering Eglantine's compliment, I thought, only a fool or me. I'm doing what they would like to do. The teachers took it as stupidity, which worked in my favour, until Brother Shear saw through me. I was, he said, cultivating 'a lazy mind', and he made me suffer with teasing questions. No doubt, I was a little diversion from stuffing thick skulls with set texts dumped on schools by unseen powers with the object of getting results. Not wanting to give him the satisfaction of proving him right, I played off the edge with speedy deflections that risked being caught in the slips, yet sometimes reached the boundary. But I was not getting away with what I wanted. Still, I thought, the end of year exams would be my revenge. I'll get the square-root of minus one in maths, and my English composition will be a blank page.

When I skipped a music lesson, my father lost patience with me for the first and last time. 'The day you stop playing the violin, boy, you'll be finished.' I tried to reassure him by saying I preferred to learn on my own. When I practised the Bach Chaconne (Partita 2), thumping out the double-stopping, he said it was like that Spanish dance performed sitting down with walking sticks.

My mother thought an apprenticeship in a haberdashery shop would suit me. She knew the family from working with the Vincent de Paul charity. If I started at sixteen I might rise to be a manager and, who knows, one day, become a partner. The prospect of a nine-to-five job dancing attendance on the town swank and fussy mothers concentrated my mind. I needed to hoist my ambitions on a more manly petard. One way or the other, I had to appear to be a serious person in my parents' eyes, a solid type who passed exams. Not merely for my own sake. I was putting my mother out of countenance with my father.

I resolved to make a serious effort at study. But where to begin? I had no idea how I had learned to read and write. It simply happened. By then I knew from my father about Hegel's precept of hesitation. That is, when wavering moves on from being an instinct to being a perception, it tells you, sod-it, something had better be done about this. Endless dithering is a dead end. And so you must take a chance and act, one way or another. Life has to be got on with (or got away with). Maybe by putting my head down, and not thinking about it, I would stumble upon trigonometry or gerunds and discover they hold no mysteries.

My days of daydreaming in the meadow of adolescence were numbered. No more losing myself in the long grass of summer, and letting my imagination run wild. No more disappearing down the disused railway line to the estuary where I would find a mossy dune and linger there for hours, counting how long the cormorants in the river would stay underwater (the record was four minutes), and wondering about girls and other mysterious creatures. To be conspicuously serious, constant surveillance would be desirable. I would have to wall myself within the confines of a room, where unseen eyes would know where I was all the time.

But sitting down to study for me was the electric chair. I died on the spot. And so I worked standing up like Hemingway, as though preparing to go out. Our family motto is *Fulminis Instar* (Like Lightning), and getting things over as quickly as possible was my aim. However, I found I could only concentrate on my books when smoking one of my father's pipes, and constructed a shelter with branches in a copse in the garden. There I puffed shag tobacco in harmony with my breathing. I inhaled my lessons sitting cross-legged on a nest of bracken. In winter I lit a fire to keep warm and roast the occasional potato. I discovered Arthur H. Mee's Wonder books in three volumes which explained everything, from the creation of the world to Howard Hughes's *Spruce Goose*. And with cartoon illustrations (germs had evil little faces and swishing tails). Although my mother no doubt saw the smoke signals, she said nothing.

The school liked me even less when I abandoned the dead bat. My eagerness to answer questions made the boys cheer rowdily at first, but I was soon put down as too clever by half. And they were right. My Wonder books' simplifications were open to correction. I took the brunt of Brother Shear's sarcasms, and learned to keep my hand down. I returned to the back of the class with the bad boys, who passed around comics and rude pictures, and fought silent battles over bags of bulls eyes and acid drops. I joined in with their skittishness, and Brother Shear, who didn't spare the leather strap, found me particularly rewarding. I took it on the knuckles, dedicating the pain to my rehabilitation back into a normal boy. Fingers still stinging, I was emboldened to thank him. 'Are you taking the mickey?' he snarled. 'On balance, no,' I said. He gave me a dark look, but the boys all laughed. I was one of them. Was I learning to forget myself with social double-stopping in order to tap applause?

However, I thought of my mother, and locked myself away with the proscribed textbooks. I could block out all thoughts of escape for the duration it took to smoke a bowlful of tobacco.

By breathing easily and spitting at regular intervals it was possible to keep it going for almost an hour. Taking my cue from Nietzsche's, 'Credit no thought not born in the open air and while moving freely about', I resumed my excursions along the shore of the estuary. This time with Longman's Latin or *As You Like It* open. Study in motion had something of the freedom that I loved when I ran and ran. The words went round and round like fireflies around a lamp bulb until they burnt themselves into the light of memory.

My mother reported the serious effort to my father, and he took me on his evening walk. I even ventured to ask his advice. Numbers were easy. They added up. But learning words off by heart and regurgitating them seemed pointless. Remembering them didn't tell me what they meant. He patiently explained that numbers didn't have to mean anything except themselves. While words mean something else. They make you think. And the more you think the more uncertain you become. But you feel your way into them and one day the original words come back, and you understand them without knowing why. He called it 'tacit understanding'.

All very well, I reflected, but waiting for the moment when the *felt* thought became clear could take forever. Hegel's precept of hesitation hadn't the time for that. I wanted what I learned to construct a bridge between me and the outside world. On crossing it I would have the opportunity to apply my knowledge in ordinary everyday life. I aspired to be my mother's son: a doer. Nevertheless, on my father's side, I knew that behind every act there was an idea and understanding it was necessary to do the right thing. I was between the devil of getting things done and the deep blue sea of thinking about it.

MY LIFE AS A SERIOUS PERSON

Despite making progress with studying, my reputation at school hadn't changed. My marks remained in the bottom half of the class. This was partly because I tended to spell words as they sounded and a counter was not allowed at exams. I wasn't bothered. Being better than reputed meant you had something in reserve when all else failed. Brother Shear concluded my school report with, 'Capable of arrogance and self-effacement at the same time.' My father was outraged. 'It is not possible to entertain two opposite characteristics simultaneously. It breaks the law of non-contradiction.' The lynchpin of Greek philosophy was sacred to him. He wanted me withdrawn from the school. My mother brought me to see the Head Brother, who said that I needed to be held back a year to be 'ironed out'. She thanked him, took me by the hand, and out on the street vented her rage. 'Maybe putting you through a wringer would do the job.' We both laughed at the idea.

I was moved to a new establishment opened by another ex-student of my father. Dr Denny's Academy was an oasis of mirages. Not least for himself. He saw it as an experiment in transplanting English public school values to Ireland. He had a doctorate on Pedro Calderón de la Barca from Cambridge and wanted, he told my mother, to give something back. Whether this had anything to do with Calderón's *soci malorum*, the sin of being born, was unclear, but the Calderón dictum, 'We are born to expiate our existence on the sacrificial altar of life,' was said, by the unkind, to be his motto.

My classmates were dunces and geniuses rejected by other schools. The teachers were helpless in controlling them. Corporal punishment was limited to canings by Dr Denny. But sending him troublemakers would reflect poorly on their principles. The teachers had been recruited from idealists disenchanted with mainstream education which, it was said, treated pupils like circus ponies. And so six of the best was a theoretical concept. The boys got on with fooling around, or quietly studying on their own.

I profited from this amiable anarchy. When bored, I wandered out of class, and down to a stagnant stream at the bottom of the garden. There I smoked a pipe and read my books, more or less undisturbed. Occasionally a swan would climb on to the bank and shake the mud out of its wings on me. The good doctor joined me once or twice. He talked at length about the advantages of the school basket. Keeping the school litter-free seemed to be a priority. From him I gathered also that my father had it in for Voltaire's 'all is for the best in the best of all possible worlds'. On days when I had a music lesson, I played jigs and reels with a mute on the bridge so nobody could hear me.

This free-range education included one-to-one tutoring with teachers of your choice. Miss Pim, who wore a watch and chain around her neck, introduced me to the rudiments of biology, and 'Devi' Devlin elucidated differential calculus using blades of grass and a coffee grinder. His analogies taught me that numbers were not just themselves. New ones could be imagined, and applied to practical problems in, say, engineering. 'If Newton and Leibniz hadn't envisaged infinitesimal surds, airplanes would never have taken off.'

But I benefited most from Tim Labrinth. He had matriculated for university but, being too young, was taking a year out in Denny's. By the stagnant stream we talked about everything and nothing. In his old school he had been always first in the class without being a swot, and was famously sheepish when asked how he did in an exam and tried to change the subject. Once he achieved full marks in maths and pooh-poohed it, saying, 'That's impossible. I didn't finish one of the questions.'

Dr Denny was so impressed by an essay Tim wrote on Leibniz's *optimisme* and Coleridge's poem 'Work without Hope' that he wanted it published in an educational journal. According to Tim, Coleridge thought that while 'Work without Hope' is 'nectar in a sieve' (you get stuck in a dead end job), Leibniz's 'Hope without an Object' means you flounder in a quagmire till you fall on your face. During the summer holidays we renewed our friendship by the sea in Myrtleville. I had a crush on a shy girl called Jill Burns who I thought nobody would be interested in, but one day I came across her with Tim leap-stepping along the rocks, hand in hand.

It was said my father lost interest in children once they started talking. When they learned to listen he took up with them again. He left pubescent egotism and growing pains to my mother. Accompanying him on his evening walk when she was indisposed, my ear was cocked to catch his every word. I could have had a real conversation with him, but I didn't know how to broach the subject of *felt* thoughts. Once he addressed the sky with a hopeless, helpless gesture, and said, 'We won't know if we have been fooling ourselves until we die.' No doubt noticing my ears sticking out between long sideburns, he changed the subject to Brother Shear's apparent contradiction in my school report, observing that maybe he had been overhasty in his judgement. 'Dogmatism is the military wing of unreason.' Three years later, I was to read in an article he wrote that summer, 'If we wish to show another that he errs we must notice from what side he views the matter, for on that side there is usually an element of truth.' By then I had an inkling of what the question should be. But it was too late.

THE HAIRY STUDENT

After my father's death, I read *Candide,* and learned from Tim Labrinth that the 'all for the best' quote was Leibniz which Voltaire put in the mouth of the fatuous Dr Pangloss. So his enemy was not Voltaire after all, but Leibniz's *optimisme.* Was Dr Denny expiating his existential pessimism on the sacrificial altar of school life? If so, he had reason to atone. His intentions were hell paved, getting the right teachers and the wrong pupils.

I had scraped into university with Tim's help (giving me the mnemonics he used as prompts). When my siblings began to have second thoughts about the fool of the family, my mother said, 'Don't encourage him. It will go to his hair.' Indeed I was building bridges with other hairy students, and fell in with the One Ball Gang, incipient intellectuals led by Congol O'Curry, a lapsed seminarian, much given to saying 'perhaps'.

The One Ball Gang dabbled in poetry. But, when they moved on to the transcendental thinking of Pierre Teilhard de Chardin, I distanced myself, and became a founder member of the Lee Road Anarchist Society (defunct after a few months as the only other member, Hugh J. Murphy, fell in love with his landlady). We were taken by William Godwin's ideas on freedom and the common good. 'Governments lock us up in institutions to save us from ourselves. Society, on the other hand, if left alone, brings out the best in people. We release ourselves to promote happiness.'

Officially I was studying medicine but, as my mother no longer had to prove herself with me to my father, I was happy to become a chronic. I was at peace with my father's memory. Rather than hacking it in a dissection room I decided he foresaw my future elsewhere. Shortly before his death I showed him an incipient poem, and he picked out a line, 'Beyond the cliff, ten thousand years of trees,' and gave me his red velveteen copy of Shelley. His love of music would be mine. Not with the violin, but with the music of words.

A poem of mine was broadcast on radio. As I was failing exams in the university, I used a pen name so my mother wouldn't know. I went to see the presenter, Austin Clarke, the poet. He was busy preparing a programme, but gave me five minutes. I thanked him for dropping the line, 'He got shot' (it was about the assassination of John F. Kennedy), and asked what I had to do to become a poet. 'Always get paid.'

My mother found out about the visit, and was not best pleased. Austin Clarke was held in high esteem in the family pantheon. His recitation of poetry on radio was second to Victoria de los Ángeles in my father's ritual listening. Nevertheless, my mother calmed down on realising I wouldn't be disgracing the family name. But, when the *Irish Press* published me in its New Writing page, on seeing the poem's title, 'Dolly Price of Bulldog Lane', I was in the doghouse again. Dolly was very much alive.

I showed more interest in medical studies to redeem myself. We were starting human dissection. Professor Mach's preamble solemnised the first incision with St Paul's, 'When I was a child I spoke as a child, I understood as a child, I thought as a child. When I became a man I put away childish things.' Then he recommended we read *Alice's Adventures in Wonderland*. He didn't appear again in the dissecting room.

Mach concerned himself more with living anatomy. At his opening lecture he showed a clip from the first movie ever made, Muybridge's galloping horse, and footage of ballet and army drill in slow motion. Mach was a reserve officer in the Territorial Army. I skipped dissection and joined the student corps like most of my classmates. There I distinguished myself at the Easter camp by dislocating my double-jointed elbow to avoid square-bashing (the joint jumped out of its socket on firm pressure). When the visiting commandant came to inspect the sick bay he saw me reading *Brighter than a Thousand Suns*, a book about the first atomic bomb, and nodded approval.

Mach duly failed me, telling my mother that I would be a safer bet playing the violin than administering to the sick. But I didn't have a choice. Love and air is for the birds. I spent the summer dissecting with the other chronics. The squeamish laughed a lot. It gave them courage. Our scalpels were guided by Dr Fitz who had ballet hands. Nothing is as beautiful as an old pauper's unclaimed corpse when subject to the skilled unpeeling of the veins, arteries, nerves and vital organs. Dr Fitz talked us through the contour map of the body, telling us that human dissection was banned by the Vatican in the sixteenth century. Descartes's ideas on the divide between the soul and the body influenced the decision. The sanctity of the living spirit rather than death's morbidity was the only proper subject for study. A bright boy asked if that meant the dissection of live bodies would have been allowed. Dr Fitz paused, and said, 'I suppose so. Holy wars had the imprimatur.'

A print of Rembrandt's *Anatomy Lesson of Dr Nicolaes Tulp* sealed my commitment to the living dead. Human dissections were public occasions in the Netherlands. Anyone could attend if they paid a tulip. While contributing to medical knowledge, the emphasis was humanist; solidarity with those that we soon would be joining. Rembrandt was commissioned to record the occasion. He catches the hushed reverence of the seance. The expressions on the faces of the doctor and his students tell you that the soul may have departed but the body still matters.

Descartes had moved to Amsterdam at the time, so that he could think more freely. Attending Dr Tulp's demonstrations changed his ideas. Witnessing the exposure of the pineal gland in the brain, the 'third eye' which alerts us to light and darkness, he saw it as where the soul meets the mind and body. Man was made whole. He turned from speculative philosophy to focusing on the natural law which insists that we must strive to ensure the general welfare of mankind:

> Knowing the power and the actions of fire, water, air, stars, sky and all other things around us, we would be able to apply them in the same way to all the uses to which they are adapted, thereby making ourselves the masters and possessors of Nature. This would enable us to savor the fruits of the earth, and all its comforts, to preserve our health. Health which is without doubt, of all the blessings of life, the most fundamental. For the mind depends so much on the condition and relation of the organs of the body. If the wisest and most practical men could be brought together in the domain of medicine the well-being of mankind would be best served. 'Man's health is his highest law', according to Cicero.

Descartes had his reservations about what seventeenth-century medicine had to offer. But predicted that with study it would become the basis of human welfare. 'Numerous illnesses would be eradicated, both of the body and of the mind.' He even contemplated the possibility of reversing 'the infirmity of old age if we had sufficient knowledge of its cause and of the remedies with which Nature is equipped'. The socio-political consequences of this did not escape me.

Mach was in America during the autumn exams, and I got an A-plus. But the following year I failed pathology twice, and had to repeat the year. 'At least your father was spared that.' My mother's voice hardened; 'You're no good.' Her disappointment with me became mine. I smoked my pipe more and studied, Hemingway-like on my tiptoes. After many a setback, and a set-to with the Faculty Dean, I was allowed to sit the final exam.

I had skimped on clinical work. It wasn't that I didn't like patients, but they made me feel I was failing them with hit-or-miss treatments, and that made me an embarrassing presence amongst the sick. Moreover, I became pale and loitering when confronting bodily fluids; a weakness that I shared with my mother. Before her marriage she started training to be a nurse, but fainted at the sight of blood. Yet the country girl in her didn't hesitate to cut the throat of the live turkey that her mother sent for Christmas. I had been at ease with human dissection. Mach had the last word on my inglorious passage through medical school. 'You would have made a good clinician for the dead.'

Professor Latham, the external examiner, liked my written papers and, after a post-viva interview, I was let through on the understanding that I would go into research rather than clinical practice. I was awarded a Bachelor of Medicine on the proviso that I did not apply for an MD (which would allow me to treat patients). And so, Descartes in mind, I was off to London to make a living in a city that Shelley thought resembled hell ('A populous and smoky city;/ There are all sorts of people undone,/ And there is little or no fun done;/ Small justice shown and still less pity'). He had tried to bring on to the streets William Godwin's idea of 'promoting happiness by eliminating guilt', and was asked to move on by the bobbies. But I reckoned that London was now too densely populated for an individual to be accountable other than to himself. I would be left alone to get on with getting away with things.

The idea of living with the ancient Irish enemy excited me too. Kierkegaard's ideal, 'Be objective to yourself and subjective to others,' would be my guide. Then I could be clinical with English people, all the better to understand them and my prejudices. I was hoping to live in peace in the domain of medicine, at the futuristic end, rather than the ancient battlefield. I would be starting at the bottom. A job as a technician in a laboratory had been mentioned in my post-viva by Professor Latham.

The Dean's parting remark was that my degree would only qualify me to do another one. I'd be in my late twenties before I could hope to find a secure corner where in demure lighting I could pass for a person serious enough for my mother to stop worrying about me.

Nevertheless, on the plane, I began a poem:

> A refugee from my roots,
> on my own for the first time,
> carrying cases tied with twine,
> bursting with sweaters and boots.

PART ONE

'You don't inhabit a country. You inhabit a language.'

—E. M. Cioran

I

NICE NOISES

'Inconsistency in feelings is the surest sign of genuineness.'

—Jean-Jacques Rousseau

MAL COMBES

I HAD A LETTER OF INTRODUCTION TO MAL COMBES, A senior Consultant surgeon, from Professor Latham. When we met in the lobby of the Royal College, I immediately decided he was my nemesis. My mother liked to say, 'the best of goods come in small parcels, and so does poison.' Mal Combes was low-sized, and had a lethal look. Without sitting down he read Latham's note, and asked for pen and paper. Writing a name and address in my pocket notebook, he said, 'Use my name as a reference,' then turned his evil eye on me. 'Quoting poetry in your final exam? Well, I never.' Peter Latham must have mentioned that in one of my papers I quoted Hilaire Belloc. He flipped through my notebook and, no doubt, noticed the jotted next lines of the plane poem ('In the city round me sing, / cauldrons of unholy loves. / Feeding peaches to the doves, / I feel free to stroke a wing.')

'I am interested in the interface between science and poetry,' I said with undue dignity.

Mal Combes laughed. '"And let us, never, never doubt / what nobody is sure about." When I told my wife about your poesie, she said we must have him for dinner. But don't be alarmed, we won't eat you. Nasty has a passion for verse and worse.'

The biomedical laboratory in the London hospital took me on as a projects assistant. I was on the lowest possible rung, but it included time off for courses and study. Mal Combes visited as he had several research studies going, and spotted me. 'Ah, the Poet,' he said. 'I may need you sometime.' And he took my phone number. 'Nasty sends her best dishes.'

It was only when I found myself living near him in Highgate that I met Nasty. Thanks to Ian Russell, the local librarian, who I had been talking to about Rilke, I had been invited to read poems at the book club. Afterwards, a larger-than-life woman with a fox fur scarf came up to me and said, 'You're Mal's poet. I'm Nasty. Come and see us some time.' That's how I was to become a regular visitor to the Combes's. Mainly to swap books with Nasty, and to talk to his daughter Una about Jung. Mal Combes saw me as a harmless diversion for his womenfolk, and took no interest in my future. We got on well in a master and dog sort of way.

The lab job didn't exist on paper. My pittance was paid from grant-support reserves, and for the first year projects were within the hospital. But nobody seemed to know what I was supposed to do. Charles Baron, the lab director, said, 'Just make yourself useful by doing nothing.' And so I became the dogsbody in a white coat who ran messages, and enrolled in a medical statistics course. The only other student was an

Irishman, Manannan O'Hickee, on an Irish government retraining programme. There was no proper supervision or formal lectures. We learned by picking the brains of those who knew the field. O'Hickee's facility with *plámás* (cajolery) made them happy. By the end of an eventful year, we knew the rudiments of research design and evaluation, and were awarded diplomas in public health.

O'Hickee was a fellow pipe-smoker, and so we studied well together. We also had beards in common, and got on in a mutually undemanding way. People saw us as the Irish Laurel and Hardy (he was the fat man, but did not fool himself). However, it wasn't all laughs between us. We were thoughtful about one another's lives. As an overseas placement he would be going back to where I belonged by birth. While I had burnt my boats. Although, since I had never felt completely at home anywhere, I couldn't truly call myself an exile. Despite his settled life in Ireland, he was a man of the world, and his sojourn abroad had made him feel young again.

Unlike the calypso that everybody was singing, O'Hickee was looking for 'experience', not 'youth'. He flirted shamelessly with every 'Mamma Jacobs that walked bold at night', face like 'Jack Palance', or not. In the Jewish sandwich bar on Ashfield Street (scene of the last Ripper murder) he told me how to please women. 'Always admire the hair. It never fails.' His admiration for the *radabarbara* who ran the place knew no bounds. The hair was not only big but it changed in style and texture from week to week.

O'Hickee's inspired flights of courtly verbal floats went down so well our apple salmon sandwiches increased in size *and* the price fell. She was clearly *stuck* on him, and fluttered when he called her Rahab, a generously proportioned woman (Ian Russell was tutoring me in Yiddish). The two talked of life on this planet in a mocking way, veering into agreeable nonsense. When I intervened to say one non-sequitur was an Irish bull, she said, 'What?' O'Hickee explained, adding in quotation marks, 'An Irish bull is always pregnant.' 'Like me,' she roared laughing.

I moved on to performing routine tests for seasoned researchers, and tidying up data collection. Charles Baron saw potential, and had me contracted out to outlying hospitals for grant-supported schemes that had for lack of planning never got off the ground. I would be the coordinator. Half my fee would go to the lab. Studies of intravenous injection techniques, and the safety of benzodiazepine as a non-addictive hypnotic for mild depression, brought me into unexpected contact with drug addicts. They were queuing up to be subjects.

Getting results was not like school. A negative outcome wasn't a failure, except perhaps for the pharmacology industry. I could see a freelance career ahead of me. If I kept away from teaching hospitals I could get away with my modest qualifications in epidemiology. But to branch out on my own, I would have to communicate with the natives, and I was still in a cultural maze and haze.

VERBAL FLOATS

Yet in London I felt more at home with myself. The people around me had no idea who I was, and this enabled me to become what I was supposed to be, without trying too hard. That's not to say I was cocksure of myself. As other people didn't know me, I didn't know them. I couldn't read them like the people in my hometown, and I had a constant feeling of getting them, or being got, wrong. This ought to have made me listen and learn. But I had my way to make, and conserving my tongue would get me nowhere.

And so I braved my fear of being inopportune, and said the first thing that came into my head. Any embarrassments caused would distract me from introspection and second thoughts. I could be whatever they wanted me to be. In the event, my impromptu sallies went better than I could have hoped. Listening is not an exact science and talking is an ephemeral art, performed in passing. What they wanted mainly was a light exchange that didn't hold them up. Nobody in London had time for anybody else. I was sent packing in the nicest possible way. And so I free-associated, and let the tongue wag the brain.

Occasionally I could see from the raise of an eyebrow or a tilt of the head that that my nonsense was less well received. The English are masters of the slighting jest. They were thinking to themselves no doubt, 'The Irish are funny.' But I have a lightness on my feet with words, and getting them wrong often inspires me to compensate with a poetical riff, a verbal float of free-associations to puzzle interlocutors. Thereby using up the embarrassment in the air, until some sort of conclusion, rhyming, or not, is reached. The tilt of the head turns face on, the eyebrow falls into a slight frown, and I'm looked in the eye. A truce has been signalled, and we can get down to business with the ordinary everyday commonplaces that make us feel good about one another, and thus advance practicalities.

From an early age I have rehearsed conversations with the talking in my head. Remarks I hear in passing are entertained

and submitted to free association until I come up with a satis-
factory response. It was only for myself, but it prepared me for
secondary socialisation. The verbal float, if it isn't to disappear
up its own air, also calls for practice. Improvising associations
with strangers, or people at one-remove is facilitated by a polite
boomerang. For instance, someone says to you, 'Odd weather
for this time of the year.' You float back, 'It's not this time of
the year.' Mutuality is achieved courtesy of a pregnant Irish bull.

I practised with friends like O'Hickee, Ian Russell or my
neighbour, Joab Comfort. I'd say what I like, and if they didn't
like it, say it again with knobs on, until they told me to shut-up.
People that don't know you are more susceptible. Alertness is
the key to making the potential embarrassment work to your
advantage. An amiable approach works best. If you keep your
head clear of unpleasant thoughts, the art of softening a hard
word or sweetening a bitter one is easier than unsticking a super-
glue solvent. It only takes a few seconds, not an eight-hour soak.

Joab Comfort lived in an apartment adjacent to mine and, as
he 'knows everything', I often sought his advice on the staircase.
Verbal floats interested him as he was studying artificial intelligence. Joab opined that, 'They're not unlike Ornette Coleman
with his buddies mugging free jazz on a homemade instrument
(stuck together with spit as Don Cherry said). Lightening the
heavy or giving the trivial gravitas is a gift common to great
jazzmen. Once the parameters have been defined, the variations
jump in to contradict them, until an accommodation is reached.
The blue notes, and compromising licks, come fast, but they have
been coming a long way. A lifetime of study and solo jamming
is behind it, and there are hereditary factors. Thelonious Monk
played an imaginary keyboard even when he was eating.'

I wanted to counter Joab's riff, but he was off before I could say that the practised verbal float is more a characteristic of the Irish leprechaun shoemaker. The little man sits at his last, with cheerful aplomb premeditating his next trope. Meet one in a wood clearing and he will not show surprise. The rather formal stutter slows things down to allow him pause to second-think you. Affability cloaks an implacable sense of himself, self-conscious but self-assured. After an encounter with a leprechaun you leave contented. You couldn't meet with a nicer little fellow. Nevertheless you soon realise you have been fooled somehow by the fairy logic of his verbal floats. You don't resent it. Fair enough. Being outwitted by a master is the comeuppance of the complacent.

SPEECH MELODIES

In order to counterpoint the verbal floats by reading the interlocutor's response, I moved on from free jazz to Leoš Janáček, the Czech composer. Joab led me to him. 'Eighteenth-century music had its ear cocked to nature. Mozart took his notation from the lark outside his window to create the motif for his first violin concerto. The twentieth century has humanised sound.'

At the *fin de siècle*, Janáček started collecting what he called speech melodies. He began notating the pitch and tempo of common speech, making transcriptions of the noise of people around him. He recorded the cries of children, the groaning of old people, the neighbours gossiping, and even, to distract himself from despair, the ravings of his daughter when she lay dying of typhus. Above all he listened to people. 'Even if I didn't grasp the words, I grasped the rise and fall of the notes. I knew what the person was like. How he or she felt. Whether he or she was lying. How upset he or she was. The speech melodies were a window into their soul.'

As my job became more serious, or rather I became more serious about it, I worked harder on inducing a two-way conversation. I concentrated on how others sounded and looked when they spoke, rather than what they said. If the other person was aware of my close attention, I found that released the Mozart's lark dimension for both of us. You could induce a more spontaneous response with a gimlet eye. A lilt or *basso profundo* in my voice, in accord with an amused interest, or frank despair at not getting what I was saying, offered the listener a cue to speak. And by gauging the intonation, and looking at what the eyes and the tilt of the head were expressing, you could read their mind. But all too often in their confusion, they ejaculated a pipsqueak 'really' and the dreaded 'let's face it' and you had to try again, patiently building up their confidence in not having to make sense, at least of the common kind. You were encouraging them to embark on a soaring verbal float of their own. A rare event but worth waiting for.

More commonly the patter rambled on with a certain complicity. The words may be going everywhere and nowhere, but by listening birdlike, nodding along with the drift, the trailing away into an uneasy silence could be prevented. It was like clapping along with the music. No one is going to stop when the audience is obviously appreciative. The patter goes on until the grounds for it are exhausted, and it's swallowed up in a babble. Or it takes to the air with a soar.

'Not all ventriloquists have dummies. Be wary of anyone who speaks through unmoving lips,' said Ed Dorn, the puppet-master poet, and I was listening to him. You hear what people are saying by trial and error. When failure stares you in the face and your interlocutor is about to walk away mystified, or scornful (depending on status, or temperament), a look of fascinated interest can reverse the loss of momentum, and he or she relents, and says any old thing to fill the gap in the air that is closing in. This is not the moment to interrupt. Something surprising can be said that is particularly important.

The point of free association is that it liberates the spirits, the daemons and angels are up in the air. As with a declaration of love, it surprises the supplicant even more than the object of it. What's blurted out may not be poetry, but being heartfelt has a grace all its own. Once a nifty finance manager, Rami Bashir, encouraged by my gimlet eye, told me that every decision at work for him revolved around the simple question, 'If I do that, will I be able to get my eight hours' sleep a night?' Subsequently, we talked of things in terms of a good night's sleep. The metaphor offered a peace between us which passeth understanding.

The people I've got on well with in my working life, my happy few, for the most part emerged out of the mist of mutual weariness of having to say the right thing. Something inconsequential is confided and, if I have the wit to catch the musical meaning, and realise it means more to them than the important matter under discussion, we move on to become friends. It is no longer necessary to watch what we say to one another. This common parlance isn't asserting that there is more to life than work, but that work is only a part of life.

'OMNIA MEA MECUM PORTO'
('ALL THAT'S MINE I CARRY WITH ME')

My life was signposted by Horace, and I wasn't travelling light. But what was in the baggage was what I felt might come in handy. If Shelley's hellfire view of London had proved hyperbolic, on the other hand any hope that I would be only accountable to myself was vain. I wouldn't be left alone to get on with getting away with things. And not only by the people I was working with. If the talking in my head is the unconscious speaking (Jacques Lacan), it made me answerable to antecedents and ancestors.

Childhood and my working days in London were a continuum, an estuary that opened into a sea of troubles. Both plunged me into the unclear waters of the everyday, the amniotic fluid of the serious life. The saddened look in my mother's eyes had persuaded me to stop running along the shore like a mad March hare and, instead, paddle in its shallows. Now as the waters deepened, and I couldn't stand on my feet any more, her steadying hand at one remove helped me to float. As I continued my studies, and held down a job, her weekly letters smiled confidence on me. But the murky spirits from the estuary of my adolescence returned in my sleep, and spilled out into my life. The talking in my head mumbled that going with the flow wasn't enough. I had to swim against the current to test the waters. Only a fool, or me, I thought to myself. But what could I do? I was born upside down, and now I wanted to be inside out.

However, I had my angelic indwellers as well as daemons. My father's preoccupation with higher things, and my mother's with more down-to-earth matters, coexisted in me, in a diluted form. She believed in honest worth in a naughty world. He thought of what was best for mankind in the worst of all possible worlds. His struggle for a better world was the classic paradox of the good man's distress: an example to everybody, and yet he doubted himself. On our last walk he remarked, as though talking to someone else, that he had frittered his life away fighting losing battles. And I well remember my mother's fatalistic expression when a colleague telephoned and he was drawn into some polemic or other. No wonder she hated phones.

My father never allowed himself to get away with anything. He took the world on his shoulders, and sweated blood. He was acutely sensitive to other people and hard on himself. But his awareness did not extend to how they saw him. Once a simple soul from the village didn't return his salutation and, deeply wounded, he returned home to ask my mother why. 'Jamesie isn't used to being treated like a normal person,' she said.

Most people's skin thickens with the years. The opaqueness spares our blushes. What dogs our lower depths is less evident. I covered my skin by growing a beard and wearing cycling shades to hide my impatience with others. But I wasn't blinkering myself. An example to nobody, I suffered doubts about my beautiful temperament gladly. At best I could be my father's Sancho Panza, and keep going towards horizons that might, or might not, exist. A better bet would be to be my mother's son. When I read Brecht's remark on Lenin, 'He was a functionary, who functioned,' my heart leaped up, and I resolved to be a pragmatist who actioned things. Or not, depending on the circumstances.

MAKING MEET ENDS

If I had my doubts about myself, hesitation never stopped me taking action. Once again the films were my writing on the wall, their plotting being hinged on Hegel's precept. It functions on the principle that the programme has a time limit. Logically the plot could go on forever. It needs a sod-it point to cut the dithering, and make things happen, for better or worse, before the deadline. The End prevents what Hegel calls a Spurious Infinity. An analogy between the workplace and the cinema came naturally to me. The main difference is a matter of lighting. In the cinema the lights come up, and down. In the office they're on all the time, and harder on the eyes, being usually strip. But, as one accommodates to sunlight when coming out of an afternoon showing, you get used to the glare by keeping your head down, doing what you wanted to do in the first place.

I wouldn't be working for a pension. The ultimate object of work for me was the practical application of an idea. Being paid off with a golden handshake was something else. I didn't think about it. When the lab boss Charles Baron was explaining to me that I would only get half of the allocation, but it would be tax-free, I interrupted him and said, 'I'm not interested in money,' and he looked at me suspiciously, thinking I wanted a better deal, or was taking him for a ride. 'Money is no consideration as long as you don't have to think about it,' my mother had said, as she showed me how to write a cheque before I left for England. 'Live if necessary on an overdraft, but make sure you have life insurance.'

Now I was privileged, not having to give security a second thought. It was a time of plenty for temporary posts that were state supported. When a job wasn't talking to me, instinctual hesitations would tell me that I had better do something, one way or another, and I would move on. Work was like going to the movies, I said to myself, only you were paid rather than paying to get in. It was possible to leave early when the plot thinned to the point of no return, or thickened to absurdity. A job was the golden goose but, if you killed it, there were others. Nevertheless, I stayed on in the laboratory, even though talking to my job was getting contentious. I was looking to freelance on the side, and thinking of cherry-picking clients from the lab list, possibly with the help of Mal Combes, who as a surgeon was concentrating on teaching and research.

After work I liked to drop into the Electric Cinema Club to renew my acquaintance with the butterfly of ambiguity. I saw Jean Renoir's *La Chienne*, and subsequently Jacques Becker's *Casque d'Or*, films exploiting for comic-tragic purposes the jealousy of the pimp for his clients. The hypocritical anguish of the *maquereau* with his *poule de luxe* summed up the working life for me. I walked out into the growing dark feeling I was premeditating the murder of my golden goose by betraying professional standards, and I would have to pay for it. I would never find work again in this town.

The lights were coming on to reveal the detritus of the Portobello Market. Rats were probably rooting in the spilt grain and cats tearing into rotten fish, and I realised I didn't have to prepare my exit with a left-handed form of human endeavour. Every job has its reasons, no matter how unreasonable they may seem. I sighed rather than laughed. On Ian Russell's advice, I was reading André Gide's last book *So Be It*, and wallowing in what he called his *tristesse ineffable* (ineffable sadness). I was feeling my way, and getting somewhere. Not where I wanted to go, perhaps. But what can you do? The tail wags the dog. I perished the thought of talking to Mal Combes. If my life was a film set, I would leave the door ajar like Jean Renoir ('You never know what might walk in').

SPOKE SONG

I continued negotiating the world with Janáček. The speech melodies spoke to my honest worth. I listened for signs of complicity. I extended them to all noises that registered in my inner ear. Sounds in the street and buildings I occupied were interrupted less and less by murmurs from the world I'd left behind. Reverberations from childhood like the whistle of a train in the night had no echo. Life went on like the city in the small hours. Loud and soft at the same time, and the soft was sometimes more audible. Halting pauses, as though the night has a speech impediment, are broken by articulated lorries rumbling from motorway bypasses. As dawn broke the noise crunched into double-stopping with shrieking harmonics. It is reassuring that silence doesn't exist. 'The deaf hear infinity,' says Victor Hugo. I was hearing the world as it is. Sounds coming from nowhere bursting into an unexpected clarity, like an emotion.

Charles Baron sensed my unrest and, removing the 'assistant' from my job title, sent me to the front line on my own. That is, projects nobody would touch. I didn't hesitate. The current might not be in my favour, but I was happy in the knowledge that I wasn't like everybody else. I took to riding my bike to assignments. A bike is almost as good as a dog to break the ice between strangers. Moreover, arriving on time was a rare courtesy in a city of traffic jams. If the project was out of London it could be carried in the last carriage of the train. My Mayday Raleigh had been discovered abandoned in a rotting shed in an overgrown vacant lot by Parsons, an artist friend of Nasty, who specialised in found objects. He fell in love with it ('The last of the real bikes, circa 1955'), and restored it to its glory. He sandpapered the rust so the chrome Rolls-Royced, stripping the paint off the frame until the original colour came through. It was the green of the first leaves on the trees, and had not lost its freshness. Veteran pedal-bike aficionados would die for it. I bought it before it was exhibited.

My Mayday Raleigh was a heavy metal charger that had a caterpillar grip on the road. Climbing hills without a three-speed was slow but steady. On the flat its progress was stately as a Flann O'Brien policeman. But it came into its own descending. With a nod to Yeats, Parsons said, 'the bell-beat of its spokes is cool.' And, indeed, winging downhill, it flapped a swan-like cadence. However, he forbade the removal of the heavy chainguard. 'It would be like giving the Mona Lisa teeth.' When the chain came off, a not uncommon occurrence on country lanes on the way to some cottage hospital, aesthetic concerns were secondary. Getting it back on blackened my fingers. Presenting myself to the director I would apologise for my dirty hands, and float, 'I have my Ordinary Madnesses, just like everybody else. I suppose.'

THE LARK IN THE SMOG

Madge Herron was a strange bird who waddled the streets of London encumbered by broken wings. She was built like a chick albatross, and her vocal range was that of a starling, calls varying from chortled warbles to alarming squawks with tender little trills in between. Ian Russell introduced her to me in Highgate Library. 'Madge is a poet.'

'And peasant,' Madge chirped.

'She never writes anything down.'

'Why should I? I'm a songster.'

But she had only one poem, and I heard it so often that I have it off by heart:

> Give me the lark before you cut it up.
> I wouldn't do a thing like that to get the music out.
> I'd rather be a scarecrow a thousand years instead,
> until a time when she is trusting
> and comes to me herself.
> Then scarce I'd pull the summer in
> to hear the singing in her head.

The Donegal lilt drew young poets. Some saw her as the Irish Stevie Smith. Others thought she spoke to the condition of the muskrat and the cabbage skunk. At heart-to-hearts in her Tufnell Park bedsit she force-fed effete young men big Irish dinners of bacon and cabbage. Afterwards they were given dogs' digestive biscuits.

I became one of her gentleman callers. None of us knew of the others. Madge made you feel her light verbal floats and heavy dinners were for you and you alone. I gathered that she was the daughter of a hedge schoolmaster down on his luck, forced to make a living as a tailor. A motherless child, she left home as soon as she could, living for a while in a boarding house in Dublin.

'I loved the life there to distraction. But it was unrequited. And it was all your fault.'

She was talking to herself, and with such fury that the crockery rattled on the table. 'And in front of my friend,' she cried out, and threw a glass on the floor. That calmed her, and she became the doomed bird of her poem, fluttering around the room, picking up the pieces, and whispering darkly about an undivulged crime. Then with a great laugh she cleared the bedsit of ghosts. 'What a baboo I am.' And, pouring me a tea, she remarked in the dulcet tones of her poem, 'Have you noticed the sobering influence of a drop of milk?'

I thought it was poetry, or great acting. Indeed, sometimes there was a coldness in her that reminded me of the servant who killed the bird in the kitchen in *Miss Julie*. I wasn't surprised to learn she had been to the Abbey acting school in Dublin. Amateur dramatics was strong in rural Ireland during the 1920s. Abbey scouts, on the look-out for natural talent, would have heard the beautiful voice from the back of the hall. 'They all talk like that in Glenties,' Madge told me. But I knew they didn't. George Bernard Shaw wanted her to be his Saint Joan. But she was already a fully-fledged lark. And her mind gave way. She disappeared into the London smog to re-emerge after the war as a char to the literary elite. 'Tear me apart for my bad verses,' Madge said, when she recited her poem at the Lamb and Flag poetry readings. She was a play within a play.

I wearied of the heavy food, and the repetitive performance, and got her to see R. D. Laing, who took her on under pressure from George MacBeth. Laing, the author of *The Divided Self*, was the psychiatrist to the poets, and wrote gnomic poems himself by numbers. Madge bad-mouthed his poetry as soulless, and he threw her out. I introduced her to Dr English, a more conventional psychiatrist, and left them to it. When I came back they were getting on so well that Madge gave him a bear hug at the door. She was walking on air. 'Isn't she wonderful?' he said. 'It would be a shame to cure her. But she's too far down the road for that.'

'Did she mention the undivulged crime?'

'Yes. In a tiny little girl's voice she said, "The sin of being born".'

'What can be done for Madge?'

'Just be nice to her. Miss Herron's trouble is she loves everybody and no one.'

When I caught up with Madge she was whooping complicity at two lovers kissing in the street. I left her to their tender mercies.

II

TALES OF ORDINARY MADNESS

'Humanity is divided neatly into two categories. Those
who want to go and those who want to stay.'

—*Yellow Lola,* Ed Dorn

NAILS

URING MY RESEARCH PROJECT FOR THE PUBLIC HEALTH
diploma, the nails of both my forefingers were mangled
while calibrating the snap power of jaws. My subjects were
patients in the local mental asylum. Their bite reflexes were not
conditioned. I resisted the temptation to bite back.

The next day I bought a metal thimble from a sweatshop in
Whitechapel. The old-world smells of wools, linen, silks, and the
threaded gold motif on the Bangladeshi tailor's apron accorded
with his courtesy. He traded my modest purchase with the same
ceremony as if I were buying the king elephant in the Procession
of the Tooth in Kandy. Although I only needed one thimble to
protect the nails, I bought one for each finger: pointillist bubbles
on the exterior and the smoothness of the Orient inside.

A few days after the bite my nails festered and the fingertips began to throb. I couldn't sleep. So I sedated myself with whiskey and with a cut-throat razor. I severed the cuticles to drain the pus until the blood flowed. I still live with the consequences of my left-handed surgery. The nail of my left forefinger splits when I'm run down. The nail on the right is a perfect hypocrite.

FIRE

In our last term O'Hickee had been trapped in a fire in the student hostel, and was lucky to be alive in St George's Hospital on Hyde Park Corner (now a hotel for global businessmen on cosmic expense accounts). The nurses wore wimples, but that did not stop him speculatively complimenting their hair. He moved from a private room to the open ward, and organised card games with miniature whiskeys as the stake. Even patients with not much to live for participated. Once when I was visiting him, he introduced me to a card cheat with cancer of the gallbladder whom he had rescued from the wrath of a posse of arteriosclerotics. Another time we contemplated a blanket covering a dead body, and he complained the man owed him three single malts. O'Hickee's corrupting influence brought pleasure into the world of the sick. His pipe was passed around, and enjoyed under the blanket. The ritual sharing out of miniatures before turning in at night brought a sounder sleep than hypnotics. The ward whistled with tipsy dreams.

O'Hickee was exempted from having to present a thesis. The examiners came to his bedside to conduct a viva on Kaposi's sarcoma in Tower Hamlets. He was generous with useless advice on mine, the bite study, but cajoled one of his smitten secretaries to type my write-up on the cheap. At my oral exam, the chairman of examiners noticed it was subtitled a *dissertation* (an 'r' was replaced by an 'n'). I was convinced it was O'Hickee's subconscious reprisal for playing him along about Rahab's hyperborean hair. Ian had told me about the *sheitel*. It was a wig so she wouldn't be a temptation to men other than her husband ('Hair is nudity,' says the Talmud).

I lost contact with O'Hickee when he returned to Ireland. A decade later at a conference in Royal College I bumped into him. I asked him about his career. 'I'm a civil servant in the Health Department. Civil to everybody and a servant to the devil' (quoting C. H. Sisson). I raised the question of the wigs, and his roar of laughter told me he knew all about it then. We talked old days, and I was surprised to hear that at the time he was grievously missing his wife and children back home. I forgot to ask him what started the fire, but I noticed he didn't smoke his pipe any more.

VOMIT

I was annoyed that Mal Combes's nickname for me had been passed on to the laboratory staff. When daydreaming at work I sometimes doodled a verse on my blotter. That would have to stop. Even if I laughed it off, I could never be one of them as a poetaster. Worse, my Mayday Raleigh was stolen. I locked it on the railings outside Somerset House, and learned too late that a pickup truck does bulk steals in central London using police belt-cutters that can cut through handcuffs. One way or another, it was time to strike out on my own with my diploma.

An evening paper had published an article about the poor attendance of ethnic families at child clinics in the inner city, and the educational consequence of undiagnosed conditions. Lambeth was specifically mentioned. Dr Thrower, the director of public health, responded with a commitment to research the reason why.

I did an O'Hickee, and cajoled the medical anthropologist, Hervĕ Thuau, to brief me. My Trojan Horse was a mediaeval medical textbook, *Rosa Anglica* by John of Gaddesden. The Irish Texts Society had just reissued it (I got a copy because when my father died I renewed his subscription). As a product of the famous School of Montpellier, the Mecca of traditional Western medicine, Thuau was delighted, and identified the various ethnic groups in Lambeth, and their marital patterns, with particular reference to family names. He was disappointed that there was no Chinese community, his latest interest. 'Traditionally the Chinese don't believe in sickness, per se, only health. Therefore attendance at preventive clinics would be contrary to custom. On the other hand, with West and East Indian and African peoples the default is no doubt due to brute ignorance on the clinics' part.' I left him feeling sorry there were no Chinese. I had been much taken by Rilke's ideas on difficulty in his *Letters to a Young Poet*. 'You must make things difficult for yourself, so that you can triumph over something worthwhile.' Thuau's flow charts on family structures and names would be enough to conclude the research before it got started.

I had never been to a formal interview before, and therefore wasn't surprised that Dr Thrower vetted applicants on his own. I had checked out his credentials. Ex-service doctor. He had retained the military moustache and air of command. Although there were no other candidates waiting, he appeared pressed for time, and impatiently tossed through my application. But Thrower relaxed as he interviewed me, or rather interviewed himself, and talked non-stop. He expatiated at length on the chaotic lives of the urban poor, concluding, 'fundamentally they are stupid. I have more brains in my arse than they have in their heads.' I waited for questions but none were forthcoming. After an interminable pause during which he tapped his paperknife on his desk, he casually remarked, 'I don't really need a researcher. I know what the problem is…'

I was stupid enough to interrupt, 'Chaotic appointments, evidently. What do reception clerks know about kinship in Afro-Asian communities? I have all the details here to provide them with an address system for envelopes.' As he leaned towards me, I found myself waving Thuau's flow charts in his face. 'I had hoped for somebody intelligent to talk to,' he growled. 'Evidently the solution is brain surgery,' and abruptly ended the interview. 'You'll be hearing from my secretary.'

She was cowering at her desk, a wee crimbly creature who took my address without looking at me.

In the rejection letter I received, an *up* was added by a stray hand to Thrower's signature.

I had it framed.

THE LIMITS OF MEDICINE

I remained on as the ping-pong ball for contracting out. Charles Baron told me that if I got publications in refereed journals, I could even hope to be contracted in, that is, employed on a regular salary. It was like saying, if I got to the Moon I would inherit the Earth. I was working with other people's ideas. I stuck to obtaining ethical approval, and progress reports. They could publish and be damned. If I didn't like the project or my clients, I would either advise abandonment, or pay a postgraduate student to do the ground work. Sometimes I found myself working for free.

Several projects were investigations into how to avoid bad medicine. Better training rather than research was what was needed. Joab Comfort insisted I read Ivan Illich's *Medical Nemesis*. Illich, the Mexican sociologist of medicine, saw the medical domain as an authoritarian conspiracy. In Roman times the Cornelian laws ordained that physicians should be punished for patient neglect or lack of skill. If the errant doctor was a citizen of any fortune or rank he was only condemned to deportation. A nobody was put to death. Formal medical education evolved from brutal beginnings. Medical practice became professionalised. Savants were distinguished from the ignorant meddlers with physic. The domain of medicine established its own order. Illich opined:

> In modern times this has led to the depersonalisation of diagnosis, changing malpractice from an ethical into a technical problem... In the 1970s in the United States less than one-fifth of every dollar paid by insurance to compensate for malpractice went to the victim. The rest was shared out between lawyers and medical experts... The medical domain with the eclipse of the explicit moral component in diagnosis has invested itself with an authority that is totalitarian.

I was not wholly convinced. Ethical committees existed. And when a proposed diet study in a mental hospital was rejected because the control group would not benefit from enhanced nutrition, it was fair enough. Nevertheless it was a good idea that couldn't be researched and proved worthwhile.

Working with others' ideas made me want to think up some of my own. One statement in Illich stood out: 'For more than a century, analysis of disease trends has shown the environment is the primary determinant of the state of general health of any population.' It married my recent training with Descartes's invocation to medical science 'to master and possess Nature (fire, water, air, stars, sky and all other things around us)'. I cycled to Broad Street and paid homage to the water pump where modern epidemiology began. Instead of working from within the medical domain, I needed to get out and hawk my freelancing in the real world. The school environment had become more open-minded with the emergence of comprehensives. And so, remembering my days as a hungry boy, I decided to propose myself to the educational authorities to review diet issues.

ON BEING DEAD BY DEFAULT

After many letters that were not answered, and one embarrassing visit to the Town Hall in Camden where the chief educational officer asked me, 'What are you trying to sell, snack vending machines?' I met a teacher in the Heroes of Alma pub in Maida Vale. Ernie was slightly drunk and wanting to talk. His wife had just run away with the PT master at the school where he was a deputy head. Ernie seemed more amused at the Mills & Boon old chestnut than sorry at his loss, except that they had taken the money collected from the children's parents for a trip to Russia. As this made him maudlin, I changed the subject by buying him a drink, and I confided my idea. The distraction proved mutually beneficial. I was able to resign from the job where I had never been properly appointed.

And so, in a tough comprehensive in a posh area of London, installed in a broom cupboard next to the canteen, I was looking into the decline in school meals. I interviewed pupils as to what they liked to eat. I didn't need to ask. When the bell rang for lunch, the pupils rushed down to the fast-food vans parked outside. Since the jobs of kitchen workers were at risk, the teachers were actively against them. I was a part of their campaign.

I questioned prowling squad cars as to the legality of pirate traders pulling up on yellow lines. The police were not helpful, saying that double parking was so widespread they could only respond to complaints specific to traffic flow. And they had their work cut out: delivery vans, stretch limos and idiot shoppers blocked bus and taxi lanes.

One hot summer's day I cycled home on my new hybrid bike for lunch to find my flat door open, and the ever-vigilant neighbour, Miss Parrish, holding my violin. It had been dumped on the steps when she disturbed an intruder. 'I've phoned the police.' The rooms were as I left them. No sign of anything else missing. So after a bite I returned to work. But there was a strike picket at the school gate, which I couldn't very well cross. I came home again.

A chunky young policeman blundered through the door, sweaty in his uniform, and refused my invitation to sit down.

'I have bad news for you,' he said and flashed a passport. 'I'm afraid your flatmate has been found dead in the courtyard of Adelaide House.'

Before I could say, 'That's mine,' the policeman fainted. He'd seen a ghost in me from the photo. Miss Parrish, who had been listening behind the door, brought him round by slapping his face.

'I'm not used to dead bodies. This was my first,' he said apologetically as she handed him a glass of water.

'What's happening?' she asked me.

'I've come back from the dead, it appears.'

Next evening a blond police sergeant called by arrangement. He smelt of graduate training college and Brut. It was his young colleague's 'first major incident'. 'Though householders are the primary victims in such cases, one must not forget police officers too have feelings.' As though it were a social call, he was looking around the apartment, and asked me if there were any similar properties in the building for sale, and roughly what price could be expected. He had a friend, etc. Finally, the PR cop left when I signed a statement that I was still alive.

The local newspaper reported that a teenager, Declan McLaughlin, had jumped from the tenth floor of Adelaide House during a police chase. The name rang a bell, and I spun my wheel of index cards. There he was, a dropout from my study, what is called a rejection. I felt vaguely responsible.

A woman knocked on my door some days later, introducing herself as the sister of Declan who died in the accident. She wanted to see the last place her brother was seen alive. I didn't invite her in, saying it was in the front garden. I forgot to ask her if Declan McLaughlin was musical.

When I think of how he died for me, I feel a little deader.

BREAST IMPRESSIONS

As Ernie's confidant I began to weary of his perpetual setbacks. The latest was that his teenage son had run away from home and joined the army. Ernie's perverse pleasure in misfortune was not mine, I thought. Communication was one-way. He had stopped listening to my verbal floats, and his speech melody was a bitter-sweet refrain, endlessly repeated. 'The world is not fair.' The only blurt of interest was that he missed the PT master more than his wife. And now he realised why she had left him. She was jealous, and avenged him by stealing his friend. But now that he had transferred his affections to me, when he offered to keep me on to work with the school doctor on a diet programme for sportsmen, I hadn't the heart to say no.

The school had a reputation for basketball. An inordinate number of very tall boys walked the corridors. The notion of being the food chain for the next Harlem Globetrotters caught my imagination. Baker Street library had an esoteric medical section, and I found an essay by Antoine Blondin about medical preparation for the Tour de France (red wine and caffeine were mentioned) and a book by Dr Pat O'Callaghan, the hammer-thrower, who won Olympic gold (1928, 1932). Despite modest means, his mother, a nurse, fed him well, and when his career was over, in the 1950s he dedicated himself to improving the diet of patients in mental hospitals. His ambition was to include sport as part of the treatment. But the Irish government, no doubt not wanting hammers thrown in lunatic asylums, vetoed any change in hospital meals.

Dr Bert was near retirement, and spent most of his time playing the piano in his consulting room. The school nurse was in despair: 'He's way behind in vaccinations.' In the waiting room the boys and girls jumped up and down to his honky-tonk. My attempts to interest this infectiously jolly man in medical preparations for sportsmen were stalled when he said, 'But, my dear chap, they're perfectly healthy,' and once again told me about 'Two Ton Tessie' O'Shea, the variety artist, who he once treated for a stomach complaint when she was performing in the Palladium. I finally realised that I was wasting my time when I found myself accompanying him on a borrowed violin in a rendering of 'Nobody Loves a Fairy When She's Forty'.

I furthered my reading of Rilke in my broom cupboard office. His concept of *schwer* (the heavy) preoccupied me. Making things difficult for yourself, so that you can triumph over something worthwhile, still appealed to me. Sometimes Rilke balanced the heavy with *leicht* (light, easy) in order to boomerang back. But he didn't find lightness easy: 'I'm heavier than gravity./ I fall, I fall without end/ to get to the bottom of myself.'

After several more false starts with the educational authorities, Mal Combes took pity on me, and introduced me to Dr Hall McCall, and his independent research unit. I was interviewed for an assistant post. Dr Hall McCall was a forensics expert with more letters after his name than anyone else on the medical register. It was said he collected degrees like embassy cars parking tickets. This time there was a panel. Dr McCall, Mrs Manders, the dentist, and her husband, Harry, who was the money (a nut and bolt factory). Mal Combes sat in as the outside observer.

The interview revolved around the gory details of an outbreak of breast biting in the posh end of Southend-on-Sea. This outbreak of neo-vampirism was threatening to top Dundee's notoriety in forensic circles as the Saturday night bottle-fight capital of Britain.

The idea of tooth prints was new, I gathered, and Dr McCall was its pioneer. My task would be to take moulds of breast bites, and attempt to fit them to plaster casts of suspects. I jumped at the job without a second thought. How could I resist such a panel: suavely condescending Mal Combes, whose confidences flattered to deceive; bullet-like Jo Manders, obsessed by detail and apparently humourless; and Hall McCall, who was said to have total recall of the future, being two steps ahead of reality. What they had in common was a certain fierceness of intent.

Dr McCall's unit had been seconded to the East Essex flying squad. He had devised bacterial tests as a sort of spit print (mapped out on a slide under a microscope and counted). Jo Manders performed them on freshly found breast bites. Though without conviction. She told me that the lactobacillus prints correlated more with the bloodsuckers' sugar consumption than individual identity. 'I ought to be doing your job with my experience of impressions,' she said, 'only Hall McCall wants to milk the Powers That Be for all the money he can get. Your post increases the miserly grant by forty per cent. You'll get half. But Harry will match it, so you won't starve. And we're hoping for a bonus from the police for every Dracula identified.'

As Dr McCall was constantly distracted by new ideas, I was left to my own devices – most of the time with a formidable policewoman, who introduced herself as 'Elly, that's what my friends call me' (though in almost a year together I didn't dare. She was always Officer Fruse). The gusto with which she took impressions of the depressed mammary glands of women in shock was a horror movie. Bloody fangs protruding over her frothing, pendulous lower lip. Or so it seemed to me. Her resemblance to the Fuseli succubus I saw at the Royal Academy was striking. The hair stood on end. I wished O'Hickee was with me. He would have called her Officer Fruse-Elly.

Matching moulds to the dental records of suspects was rarely possible, Jo discovered. Many of the suspects were vagrants, ex-jailbirds or mental-hospital patients, and the few teeth they had were loose. Dr McCall, who had old salt's blood as an ex-naval doctor, called it the scurvy factor. But Jo Manders diagnosed it as Vincent's infection, better known as trench mouth. 'It only exists now amongst the lowest of the low,' she said. Her disillusionment gave way to sarcasm, and she remarked to Dr McCall that the only decent tooth prints that could match the Johnson's Forensic Odontology Index would be from breast bites due to the prolongation of breastfeeding into adolescence. His weary nod told me Dr McCall was thinking of something else, and sure enough, he took my hand with the broken nail, looked me in the eye and said, 'Have you ever thought of taking your fellowship?' I explained that I didn't want to study any more. 'Fine,' he said. 'We start next week. I'll get you through it without study.' And he did.

Dr McCall must have passed every exam open to him and was diversifying into degrees by proxy. I was his lucky surrogate. He had obtained all his degrees in Scotland, where his ancestors came from. There he knew all the examiners, what they wanted to hear and how they decided who was fit to be a fellow. I learned more about their quirks, foibles and family life than anything else. For instance, the terrifying Professor McDuff, who had the highest failure rate, had fathered four fine boys. After dinner parties they were thrown the leftover bones to demonstrate McDuff's theory that jaw development was acquired through rigorous exercise rather than inherited. The boys all had lantern jaws like their father, and chomped through the bones like barley sugar. 'Bones are bones,' Professor McDuff proudly concluded. 'You can build them up to grind them down.'

'But it is more parental willpower that they are proving,' Hall McCall sighed.

The first viva in Glasgow tested Dr McCall's experiment with me. Professor McDuff handed me a bone and said, as predicted, 'What is that?' I replied (as instructed), 'A bone.' He didn't pay much attention to my answers after that. I had passed the one true test of a professional. State the obvious with aplomb. It's only a matter of making a virtue of the inevitable, and achieving it.

Following Dr McCall's initial success with me, I had the good sense to take Mal Combes's advice and not hazard the second part of the exam, which was clinical. Half a fellow is better than none, and enough for a freelance epidemiologist. In any case, Dr McCall had other fish to fry and cats to skin, and merely said when I showed him my certificate, 'I have a mouth-watering idea that might interest you, my half-fellow. Talk to Jo.'

THE GOOD SPIT PROJECT

Jo Manders swore by spittle. 'A film of it is what retains false teeth in the mouth. Lick it on and nature will do the rest,' she said. 'The older the patient the more superior the glue.' Jo Manders told me she first met Dr McCall at an autopsy of the unclaimed corpse of a woman dragged from the river, and being both short sized they had to stand on tippie-toes to reach the mortuary slab.

They soon saw eye to eye in more ways than one. Jo Manders told him, 'The secret of life is in saliva. Its floral composition improves with age, and if you live long enough it perfects itself, and in theory you could live forever.' The simplicity of the idea brought Hall and Jo together. Still, how was it to be tested? His ideas on auto-immunity were ahead of their time, but he lacked the technology. And so they concentrated on longevity and false-teeth retention, measuring the salivary flow and viscosity in long-livers. Hall devised a graduated sneeze test to gauge at what scale the teeth fell out. According to Pascal, 'The sneeze reflex absorbs all the functions of the soul.' I had to assume denture retention was one of them amongst the immortals. Sponsorship was obtained from the manufacturer of a dry-mouth spray. Though the company's best interests would be the other way round if Jo's theory was proved right. I was to coordinate the study.

I scanned the newspapers in the Home Counties for centenarians receiving congratulatory letters from the Queen. Two out of three were woman. Jo approached them and offered them new dentures free. Refusals were rare, the relatives made sure of that. Hardly a week passed without Jo's photograph figuring in a local paper with the fixed smiles of the longest surviving people in the land ('Long in the tooth? Not any more!'). Almost the only oldies that slipped through my net were those who died between the letter announcement and Jo's phone call to the next of kin. New subjects more than replaced drop-outs due to death. Over a year the numbers were sufficient to apply statistics to represent the degree of denture retention in the hundred-plus population in the south of England. The snuff-induced Hall McCall test showed that their false teeth withstood a force-nine sneeze, while in the control group, half their age, it was five.

Jo Manders's own spit was decidedly viscous. When she got fed up with people, which was quite often, her spitfire rarely missed the eye. It was said she inherited her sharp tongue from her mother, who lived in Last's Resting Home on the North Circular Road, and was due her Queen's letter. Jo was in two minds about making Haddie new teeth. 'Not because we hate one another, which we do, always have. But the grip of the old vulcanites she wears is incredible. Vulcanite is what horses' bits used to be made of before the space age brought in high-impact plastics. You'd need a tug of war to wrench them out. The old bitch has the fiercest spit in town, and I don't want to be at the end of it when Haddie says she wants her old ones back. She's not going to ruin my old age as she did my childhood.' Mal Combes joked that Jo was the dead spit of her mother. He wanted me to withdraw from the project, having other ideas for me (a survey by questionnaire of his pain-clinic clients).

Unlike Pavlov, Jo was not taken seriously. Just as well, as he stopped maddening dogs and experimented on people considered mad instead. She did not please her sponsors when her study disclosed that the salivary flow in her oldies was average, and so dry-mouth sprays wouldn't be needed. The sponsors asked for an explanation as xerostomia is usually age-related. Unfortunately, I had not questioned the subjects on their medications, an oversight I wouldn't be telling Jo.

Behind her back, but with Hall's approval, I subsequently used residual funding to pay the subjects for a sub-study into the control groups' drugs. Dry-mouth is most commonly a consequence of nerves. And I considered you'd need strong ones to survive a century in this evil world. The French say, 'Merde et courage, mon ami, mouiller le palais' (wet your palate, my friend, and get on with it). I interviewed each subject with a member of the family present. Their joint information confirmed my hunch. Nervous conditions weren't a part of their make-up. On the other hand, the control group wouldn't answer the question straight. They were vague about their medication, and I couldn't ask them straight out if they had a history of mental illness.

I realised that by not working within the university I had missed out on the sharp eyes of colleagues. Hall McCall's only commitment to the study was to the sneeze test once his immunity idea proved unrealistic. I tried to publish our results, but Mal Combes turned out to be one of the journal's referees. He rang me. 'Why didn't you come to me and I would have saved you the time? You let me down on the pain-clinic survey for this?' He slammed down the phone (it's not the mal in Armalite that worries me but the mal in Mal Combes). Chastened, I knew I would have to take the road to Canossa, that is, eat humble pie. I would be reined back in. I didn't doubt the laboratory would take me back. But it would be on my own terms, not Charles Baron's, I said to myself. The talking in my head was not convinced.

So Jo and I were to keep the secret of life, or at least a long one, to ourselves. We didn't trouble Dr McCall with our failure to get published. He had moved on to something else as usual: a study of tooth loss and ageing in rice rats. I was given the task of establishing the subjects' life expectancy. But the rats aborted my endeavours by eating their young. Not a unique subterfuge with laboratory animals only two generations from being wild. The rice rats were handed over to Dr Jack in the Psychology Department.

It was to be Hall McCall's farewell project. His cleaning lady had found a cache of plaster models of breasts in his wardrobe and alerted the police. He was rapidly cleared. But not every-body believed that he wasn't some sort of pervert. The *Southend Courier*, who had scooped the original story ('Hun Vice Rife in Southend'), ran one on how the university had suspended McCall for stealing research materials. The denial from the provost took a month to appear. When he retired in the mid-eighties a Scottish university gave him an honorary degree, his last.

I did write a light piece for *The Probe*. If some day it's found in the archive of unpublished submissions, the secret of life is safe. My conclusions were modest: accept your madness, stay off the drugs and the saliva will flow so you can keep your appetite up and dentures in.

Jo Manders left a file with me. 'It's about the focal infection scam that made dentistry a respectable profession and rich den-tists a byword for the opposite. And there's an account of my first job. "Focal" is for *The Pulse*, and "Dentures in the Trees" for *The Probe*.' The scrawl in green longhand with red glosses intimidated me, but I plucked up the courage and found, between the rants and scorn, some factual information and a cameo of the young Jo.

The two pieces essentially told the same story. The association between focuses of infection and mental illness still lingered in backward medical minds. Jo was employed by Dr Jebb, an ex-army psychiatrist, to extract all teeth from patients in an asylum and to make them plastic 'wallies' (false teeth resembled the standard wall tiles in post-war council tower blocks). And come the autumn, when the courtyard trees that darkened the ward shed their leaves, rosary beads of dentures hung from the branches for all to see.

I finished the sentences, restored chronology to the narrative, deleted all references to her mother, and sent it to her. She didn't reply. The last I heard of Jo Manders was that her Ferrari was still to be seen tearing through the streets of north London. Nobody could see her behind the wheel.

IDLE HANDS

I revisited Hervě Thuau, the medical anthropologist. I had forgotten to tell him about Dr Thrower (Up). He put me in contact with Dr Sufi, a genial Pakistani whose thesis was in broken English. I sidelined by helping him rewrite it. The quality of the research was passable, but when Dr Sufi came to a significant result, he was prone to rhapsodise: 'The men of the Punjab are proud, the men of the Punjab are strong…' I let him have his chest-thumping as a footnote with a faked reference.

At a loose end, I resumed reading Rilke, but I wearied of his trying to get to the bottom of why he made things difficult for himself. And so I moved on to philosophy. I was in the mood for Schopenhauer and philosophers who expressed their ideas in aphorisms, or what would now be called tweets. I found late Schopenhauer's sell-out to *optimisme* Panglossian. But I danced with E. M. Cioran, a Romanian exiled in Paris: 'I drift through life like a streetwalker in a town without pavements.' But such 'tinker shuffles' got wearisome; a skip and a jump that led to a 'so what'. E. M. himself tired of his own ingenious auto-derision, and craved 'a strong dose of banality. There is nothing more unbearable than the monotony of the out-of-the-ordinary.'

Joab recommended Michel Foucault's *The Birth of the Clinic*, and Ian Russell gave me Antonin Artaud's *Letters to My Doctor*, but serendipity intervened. A biography of Nikola Tesla fell into my hands, literally, while groping in the upper shelves of Highgate Library. I read everything I could find in Senate House Library on the Serbian who had not only pre-empted Edison in discovering electricity, but anticipated cyberspace and the world wide web.

I had found a way to get back to the laboratory on my own terms. Laboratories were entering the computer era, hesitantly, and I offered myself to Charles Baron on a freelance basis as a go-between between students completing their doctorates and IBM. He agreed without hesitation. It was a task nobody wanted. The terms would be the same as before for piecework. In effect I was back where I started.

The computers were still room-size, and came with an expert in a suit. Time was of the essence. The student only got access to the computer for a day, which usually became a night. I paid them dawn visits, and if the unfortunate hadn't reached 'results and conclusions', that was it. Back to crawling on the floor sorting data by hand.

Machines in general, like toys in my childhood, didn't interest me. But computers held no fears once I realised I didn't need to know how they worked, only what they could do, if asked nicely. They were obedient monsters, and keeping them on your side wasn't difficult if you found the right words. Joab was already using them for his work and said they were the future that had already happened.

Indeed, the payment of doctors and dentists was now fully computerised. I visited the Reimbursement Board with a project in mind. Overtreatment was in the air, particularly for dentists. The tabloids called it fraud. I thought it could also be bad surgery. It would be possible now to identify repeated treatments on the same tooth or brain with a simple programme. I knew the reasons for recurrent operations on the major organs would be controversial. So by concentrating on more routine operations – for instance, on hips and wisdom teeth – it would be feasible to separate the chaff from the wheat. I shared my idea with Edna Gray, the director. A decoder during the war, she had worked at Bletchley Park with Alan Turing. Engaging her in conversation about Nikola Tesla proved to be my password. Over coffee and biscuits, I filled her in on his personal life.

On proposing my idea to the Medical Council I got an immediate reply, saying, in effect, mind your own business. Edna Gray, being a former Serving Sister, said she would get on with it anyway ('Nobody needs to know'). However, I received an abrupt phone call from Mal Combes warning me off. 'You're out of your depth. And if you sink I can't save you. Everyone will think I put you up to it.' Once again, he didn't call me Poet, so I knew his wingspan would be folding.

PLAYTIME

Charles Baron used me for more and more menial tasks. Such as counting and classifying patients presenting at casualty. I paid the porter and nurses to do the night shift out of my own pocket. I remembered advice given me in my college days by a kindly histology technician called Flaherty. 'Don't fight your work.' I swallowed my pride, and entered into the spirit of being the Cerberus at the entrance of Hades. After all, I had been taken on originally as a dogsbody.

Paying for my night's sleep kept me awake. I thought of writing plays like in my student days. This time with some experience behind me I would base it in a sanatorium dedicated to treating people for the disease called sanity. I used a Dictaphone to get started, castigating normal human behaviour. I called it *My Crap's Last Tape*. The talking in my head lost its balance, and became personal. I raved against my Irish compatriots in London, still perpetuating the sins of their fathers, and their mothers' prayers, building underground tunnels, blowing up innocent bystanders in the streets, attending Sunday Mass and taking the sacraments. No loud-mouthed play of mine could compete with that. I stopped the recording when the babble became a blanket scream. Coming to my senses, I knew there wasn't anything I needed to dramatise. The world was as it is, incurably itself.

I kept my head down, and got on with getting on in a small way. My lowly status deceived to flatter. People knew me now, and I was called on to do more interesting tasks that nobody wanted to do. I had just enough to live on, and a modicum of freedom, which, after almost four decades on the hoof as a running boy, habit had reduced to routines. My only responsibilities were to the law, moral and civil (I tried not to lie to myself, and kept to the straight and narrow cycling lane). The enlightenment of my generation, such as it was, was entering dark times. The free spirits, having exhausted their virtues and vices in the sixties, were becoming like their parents. First marriages breaking up, alimony, children demanding attention. Idealism, put on the backburner, lost its fire. The last flicker of it was spent looking after themselves. They jogged and made sure their children took honey rather than sugar. These were my thoughts. I knew my blanket scream would only be heard by the converted in abandoned warehouses, squats or disused churches, and most of them were middle-class dropouts. So I continued on because

I had begun, like Dr Johnson's drudge, half-heartedly mugging my verbal floats and listening to speech melodies, free-jazzing a murky career with neither magnitude nor direction.

DEATH AND DISASTER AND A NEW WIFE

A by-blow of the casualty project was that I became the secretary of a sub-group to regulate urgency cover. While preparing for it I received a memo from Roger Toussaint, the roseate-faced consultant in Accident and Emergency: 'Sorry, I was unable to attend the Mortality and Morbidity Committee meeting on August 1st because two patients died in resuscitation.'

Roger Toussaint lived on the cutting edge of disaster; his clinics were reservoirs of human frailty – domestics, brawls, attempted suicides, road rage. Peak time was Saturday night. Wiring jaws, stemming blood vessels, drying out drunks, keeping the crazies and homeless at bay. The Notting Hill Carnival was his heaven and hell. It coincided with my study of outpatient attendance. I got sucked into his maelstrom. It was all hands on deck in a sinking ship. I learned how broken heads were glued and put in a halter, fractured joints were pinned together, and how to plaster broken bones.

Above the chaos Roger was the animating Godhead, ener-gising his all-too-human emergency team. Heavy duty reigned. Nothing was taken lightly. Pauses in the storm were broken by his high-pitched voice issuing fresh distortions of previous instruc-tions. He was a whipper-upper of purposeful panic. Cards were thrown up in the air, and when they fell to ground, his staff were expected to triage them into a pack for him to cut. Morning-after post mortems were like magistrates' court hearings in which everybody, himself included, was the accused. Anticipating the worst called for careful planning based on learning by your mistakes. On quiet days Roger fomented his own personal disasters by badgering colleagues and administrators about problems that only he could see. Indeed, his reputation for imagining problems was such that his urgent memo on sewerage leaks from the toilets into the storage vaults for patients' records was ignored by the hospital manager until it was too late.

Only with major disasters, like a rail crash, or a terrorist bomb, or a hurricane, was Roger calm. Nothing being left to chance, when the real thing struck it was no surprise. Appearing on television, plumply reassuring, he speaks to catastrophes like a matador to his bull. His flying squad on the ground is in control, steering the worst into the mainstream so it's swept into the Thames estuary to be swallowed up in the Channel.

Roger was not so much a disaster waiting to happen as a happening waiting for disasters. Each major one, it was said, occasioned a marital rupture – a new disaster, a new wife. He waited for them with open arms.

MAL COMBES REDUX

I didn't hear from Mal Combes that summer. But one November evening he rang. 'Poet, I want you to do something for me. I'm entertaining Vietnamese doctors at the Gay Hussar. Could you possibly pick up Una from the Edinburgh train at King's Cross?'

I knew what he was saying: if you save my skin with Nasty, I will forget your two-timing me with Edna Gray.

'Come to dinner next Sunday. Eight sharp,' he added ('It's the Mal in *normal* that frightens me,' O'Hickee used to say).

'Yes' to Mal Combes meant submission, and I could be sure his invitation had an ulterior motive. 'What next after Una?' I thought, and accepted. Apart from being curious, my murky career was drifting.

'I'm your lift, Una,' I said, and took her luggage. She was being pestered by a down-and-out. He was too drunk to express himself in words. I could see from his cigarette that all he wanted was a light. I gave him one, and he staggered down into the bowels of King's Cross. Una's interview suit sagged on her. Another opportunity to get away from her father gone awry, I thought.

Traffic was flowing freely, and driving past the Tube station I saw black smoke coming out the entrance. 'The Pope is dead,' I said. Old jokes never die. Una was too self-preoccupied to get it. Nobody would guess that thirty or so people (the exact number was never quite established) were burning to death inside. A fag-end stubbed into rubbish at the foot of a wooden escalator started it.

Una didn't speak until outside the family mansion in Highgate. 'By the way, when Nasty asks, who am I supposed to say picked me up from the train?'

'Your dad, of course, and he returned to his guests.'

The following weeks Dr McCall and Jo Manders were kept busy doing forensic tests. One of the bodies was never identified.

AXEDENT

Mal Combes changed the venue for the Sunday dinner at the last minute. Things cannot have been going well at home, I thought.

In a dark corner of the Spaniards Inn, the armpit of Kenwood House, we were like two conspirators. In the shadow around us the adulterers of Hampstead were making their arrangements. The something he wanted me to do for him was top secret.

And so I found myself entering the former Samaritan Hospital in Soho. You passed the Marie Stopes Family Planning Centre on your way down to the basement to get to the victims of torture. The rest of the building was sealed off. Our clients were mostly Somalians. Newly arrived, they did not speak English, but they smiled a lot.

Mal Combes made it clear I was a fallback for this project. Nobody wanted to do it. The object was to establish a pattern in torture techniques deployed in East Africa. The Powers That Be wanted a 'bona fide' grid for asylum seekers. A pattern, it was thought, would exclude cases of tribal branding and self-laceration. It seemed to me unlikely that anyone would go to the trouble to mutilate themselves in order to stay in England, and tribal branding could sometimes be a form of torture, but Mal Combes had been allocated the head and neck and I wasn't going to stick mine out.

The protocol said that direct contact with clients would make objectivity difficult. In any case it wasn't necessary. Since most soft tissue damage would have healed, we worked from X-rays. The evidence would be black and white. Thus relieving us of what would be considered an emotional experience.

Non-accidental injuries to the mouth and genitals were most common. Eyes were untouched. 'So they can see what is happening,' it was said. My job was identifying bone anomalies and foreign bodies, a mechanical task. And so when I had time on my hands I wandered into the waiting room. I got to know the pleasingly long-limbed Somalians, at least enough to exchange smiles. They were more relaxed than the other refugees I had come across over the years. Possibly because they carried in their persons evidence that would make it impossible to send them back.

Nails imbedded in the upper jaw were a particular speciality, and when I suggested that perhaps they ought to be extracted, Mal Combes said, 'Unless they are superficial, or infected, it is better to leave them alone. The bone thickens around them. It's the Phineas Gage phenomenon. He had a four-foot metal bolt stuck in his brain, and survived with half a face and an open brain for nearly thirteen years. The Barnum and Bailey circus exhibited him. No. Our subjects will only feel the nails when it's extremely cold, and then just a brief shock. Above all, I doubt if removing the evidence would do anybody any good.'

'Why aren't there any children?'

'They don't carry information.'

'But one would think that threatening children would be a good way of getting it.'

'Undoubtedly. But maybe the threat works, or the little ones don't survive.'

I had to force myself to smile as I passed through the waiting room.

An interpreter brought me an X-ray of a lower jaw with an axe stuck in it. It was in the possession of a gangly Somalian, who stood by smiling proudly, as though I was being made privy to a family snapshot. There was what looked like a tree trunk studded with nails in the background. The image was more like a work of art than a piece of medical evidence. A radiograph would not show up a tree, of course. The victim was clearly dead and nailed to something.

'Where did you get this?' I said to the Somalian, who spoke through the interpreter, his eyes avoiding mine.

'Who are you to ask?'

'If you don't know who I am, why are you showing it to me?'

'He says it wasn't him but me,' said the interpreter, 'which is true.'

'It's not right playing games with torture.' I spoke too loudly. 'It's bad enough as it is.'

They talked together in a tongue that seemed to me like arcane poetry, euphonious but harsh around the edges. I listened, nodding my head, bowing slightly, sorry I had shouted, until the Somalian began to smile again.

The interpreter explained that the X-ray had puzzled all the doctors in the detention centre, and his client had thought I might be able to throw some light. He had picked it up in a market in Mogadishu.

Mal Combes laughed, 'A piece of contemporary archaeology. The Third World often throws up strange things. It's probably an artefact produced by trick photography. But, I think, you should move on. Hanging around here is not for a poet.'

There was a rumour circulating that a member of the team had been approached with a bribe to swap X-rays. Could Mal Combes have considered me a soft target for the asylum seekers? I saw my part of the work through to spite him, but avoided the waiting room. I found I could no longer smile.

Mal Combes was thoughtful too. He invited me around to his house to discuss the work. I was embarrassed and found myself explaining Hegel's precept of hesitation. He cut me short, and I learned that the Home Office had assured the Department of Health no action would be taken based solely on the forensic evidence. But asylum seeking, he said, is a political football, and the rules of the game are ambiguous, being made as the popular mood takes them.

Ambiguity this time reared an ugly head. In the cinema of my youth it may have seemed like a butterfly settling on the floral audience, but in politics it was more like a hornet's nest. Mal Combes was less fanciful. And murmured darkly that one must never underestimate the power of grey areas. No more was said.

III

TALES OF
EXTRAORDINARY SANITY

'Life is a piece of string and love is the knot.'

—Anon

FEEDING THE GRACES

I SPOKE TO DR JACK, MY PSYCHOLOGIST FRIEND FROM HALL McCall's farewell experiment. He took his holidays by working with widows and orphans in war zones to get away from his 'well-heeled clients'. 'Think of the victims of torture that don't get here,' he said. 'Yours are amongst the lucky ones.'

I dropped in on Mal Combes at the weekend and we talked. He didn't agree with Dr Jack. 'The dead don't suffer.' 'Except in hell,' I floated and bit my tongue. His righteous anger was heartfelt. He took me by the arm into the junk room to see an oil painting. 'When I was a young man like you I painted this house, and over the years I painted myself into it,' he said wistfully. The picture was as schematic as an architectural drawing, except for a rather wan figure in the foreground, looking into the house, and finding nobody at home. 'It's a still life,' Mal Combes said sadly. Then, recovering his usual aplomb, he steered me into the kitchen to 'demonstrate how a master surgeon prepares a green pepper for the pot':

'Cut the root out with a potato knife. Peer into its interior.

'The seed formation is never the same.

'Nothing in life is as perplexing.

'Specialists pick out the seeds individually.

'Consultants nip the top off and run the tuber under the tap.

'A poet would stare down the abyss of a pepper for all eternity. But we surgeons know all about your precept of hesitation and say sod-it.' He slashed the red pepper into pieces with a fine knife. And, potting them, groaned, 'Una.' He fell into a silence so profound that it was as though his thoughts were boiling inside the pressure cooker. As the pot let off steam he ricocheted with relief. 'What Una needs is an older man to settle her.'

I was almost family now. Mal Combes took me to afternoon tea in Fortnum & Mason's with Nasty. She was looking her best, a big, handsome woman. I could see why Una had problems with her young men. Mal Combes was grimly listing eligible husbands for Una. Nasty had something horrible to say about each. What they had in common was middle age, plenty of money, confirmed bachelor status, and a mother recently deceased, or put in an old people's home. Mal Combes maintained that a made match would be ideal for Una. She wasn't getting any younger. The best she could expect was a solid type who wouldn't beat her. 'So much for love,' said Nasty.

'Love never made anyone happy,' grunted Mal Combes. 'At least for long.'

Nasty laughed, 'So much for me.'

I quietly intervened: 'Happiness according to the philosophers is an amateur concept. What does it mean to you, Master?'

'How should I know? "I'm-so-happy" is something someone else says without thinking.'

'That sounds like a happy thought to me,' said Nasty.

'Or a line from Cole Porter.'

But Nasty was distracted by the next table, and nudged Mal. 'Oswald,' she cooed, and in the whisper of a thistledown parachute spiralling explained to me that he was the spiritual leader of a get-happy cult that prompted Una to dump Tony Nakache, the orthodox accountant who wore a suit and trilby at the seaside. Oswald, a bald Antipodean with an open-neck shirt and a talkative Adam's apple, was sitting with three young women. I wondered if his complexion – a blush that did not blanch – came from supping on the blood of virgins. Oswald fed the young women tidbits of Eccles cake from his plate. I wondered if diet control was his secret. Nasty read my thoughts: 'Una is losing weight.'

Mal Combes was looking at Oswald with hate. 'That brain-scoop twisted her mind against me.'

'Now, now, you know that's not true, Mal,' said Nasty, 'Una had to get away from her depressing friends and you-know-who. And Oswald behaves like a perfect gentleman. He introduces her to serious young men.'

'A fat lot that will do her.'

'Or them. But she's perfectly happy.'

'Even you know that that's not true.'

'It's all green peppers to me,' I said. The widening marital gulf needed a verbal float.

'Shut it, Poet, you're beginning to dribble.'

'What is happiness?' I said, getting back to where we started. 'More to the point, what is love?'

'Yes, do be quiet,' said Nasty. I had reunited them.

Oswald kissed Nasty on the cheek on his way out, and shook Mal Combes's clenched fist. The three Graces threw kisses.

'What a nice man,' said Nasty.

'What a brain-scoop,' said Mal Combes.

'Poor Oswald and the girls. All in love with the same man.' Mal Combes and Nasty looked at me strangely.

'I'm just quoting what Katharine Hepburn said about Warren Beatty's women. It was the first thing that came into my mind.'

Mal Combes shrugged his shoulders, and Nasty regarded me with regret.

You could stare down the abyss of a green pepper for all eternity.

MY MURKY CAREER

I paid a hurried visit to a retired undertaker who lived in the basement flat below me. Some weeks after his wife died he had sent me a letter. Two phrases were underlined in gothic ink:

Dear Sir,

I received your note this morning. I suppose you are troubled just now in a different way from me but still troubled. I can't type and I can barely write and I am so nervous of being alone.

However I hope to see you at the time arranged.

Don't mention the suit if you are not interested. For you or one of your friends. I shall understand. My late wife bought it for me as a surprise on my last birthday... I couldn't wear it. In fact I break down when I look at it. I can't describe my feelings. I can't never get over this *body blow*.

Yours respectably,

C. B. Osbourne

P.S. I would sell the suit for fifteen pounds which is *giving it away* but it will help to pay the funeral account.

I declined to sit down, and stood there twiddling in my impatience, not wanting to be late for an appointment. I made nice noises, telling Mr Osbourne he could knock at my door anytime, but didn't mention the suit. I declined his offer of a collection of old pipes. 'They're a free gift,' he called out as I left, wondering what he meant by me being 'troubled'. My note to him had been merely polite.

The appointment was a meeting set up by Mal Combes. He was on the tail of a vaccine for the killer hepatitis B, common amongst drug addicts and their associates, and a serious danger to medical staff and therefore patients. In order to test the vaccine, he had obtained antibodies from the army in South Africa, where the virus was rife, and put together a team of fast servers. I was brought along as a ball boy.

The eminent Stanley O. Kay in the chair prefaced the meeting with a learned caution: 'The superstition around vaccines has reigned in England since the eighteenth century, even amongst the enlightened.' And he defined what he called the emperor principle: 'The ideal vaccine is one that everybody receives, except yourself, and so you are protected without incurring any of the inconveniences or risks.' Mal Combes was impatient with

Stanley O. Kay's ironies, and interrupted him, saying, 'Old chap, your history of medicine is eagerly awaited.'

My task was to find subjects from high-risk groups to test the vaccine. But social and health workers were wary. African blood was said to be riddled with a new pox. It had something to do with aid workers and monkeys. I came up against the emperor principle everywhere I went. In despair, I played the life-and-death emotional card with potential subjects, and that put them off even more. Under extreme pressure from Mal Combes I produced a handful of junkies from a rehabilitation centre where Ernie was friends with the director, and two tattooists of dubious hygiene from Notting Hill Market, who wanted the money.

Mal Combes was not impressed. He got someone else to round up London-based students from Botswana where the disease was endemic. But procrastination put paid to Mal Combes's ambitions. At the Middlesex Hospital Dr Dane's team came up with a vaccine, which apparently had been tested on the relatives of carriers. It was the nearest I was to get to the Nobel Prize in my murky career.

Mal Combes said nothing to me, and a few weekends later I braved dropping in to see Nasty and himself. 'Poet, I have something I want you to do. Take a holiday, a working one. I understand cases of cancrum oris are to be found in depressed towns along the São Francisco River in Brazil.' Cancrum oris was a condition caused by extreme malnutrition in infancy. It was so rare in the developed world that surgeons would operate free of charge. Mal Combes would arrange this.

I had just seen Romain Gary's *Les oiseaux vont mourir au Pérou* at the Electric Cinema Club, and the thought of a flight to South America excited me. But my escape to Brazil was not to be, for the time being. An Oxfam worker reported that the sightings were a hoax. A doctor in the outback, hoping to tap into First World money, had withdrawn the claim, under pressure from the government. I took a trip to the London Library instead, and read Claude Lévi-Strauss's *Tristes Tropiques*.

Lévi-Strauss was my age when he wrote his masterpiece, having abandoned fieldwork in anthropology, and taken to philosophy. I asked myself, what have I done to justify my existence? I had got away with a low-achieving childhood and, despite my pathological self-consciousness, managed to make a modest living by opportunism and luck. But, unlike the running boy that I once was, I hadn't an idea in my head, beyond immediate functional requirements.

I dropped in on Nasty to talk about books on Brazil, and Mal Combes broke into our conversation to say, 'Poet, stop this conceptual backpacking. You need to retrench, and think seriously about what's left of your future. You haven't yet found a point of application in life, and your gay abandon is beyond its sell-by date.' He loped off looking pleased with himself. Nasty laughed, and remarked, 'You spend so much time in the cinema, maybe you should become a projectionist. But what Mal says is true. You're not as nifty on your feet as you once were.' Nearing forty, I knew it was time to put away childish things, turn my back on the hustlings, and take on a real job. If possible, a useful one with a large idea behind it. I resolved to become my father's son, in a small way.

THE LORD OF THE PANOPTICON

I lingered in the London Library, enthralled by the seventeenth-century French philosopher, Claude Brunet. I had found an uncut copy of his *Pensée Solitaire* in the vaults. He went beyond Descartes's *cogito ergo sum*, and Berkeley's things-exist-because-I-think-them, to advocate absolute solipsism. He described a kingdom, Panopticon, where the world is seen in its entirety though through a glass darkly. It has a king and one subject and they are one and the same person. What he sees is the idea behind what is beyond: for example, the idea of pots and pans, bread and butter, bodies and feelings, horizons and lakes, mountains, seas and skies, and the idea of ideas, old and new, right or wrong, good or bad, resolved or incomplete, imagined or forgotten. The King rules over himself with no ulterior motive except to idealise things and possess the idea in his mind. His kingdom is not a clearing house or a power base, or a waiting room. There is no inner sanctum, or outer manifestation. Nothing happens, everything is in the head. You think, you live. You live to think.

Disappearing into the world of ideas while slumped behind smoked windows I knew was hopeless if I was to make something of my life. The dark glass had to be shattered to reclaim the reality from the idea and harness the possibilities to *get things done*. In other words I needed to get out more.

I paid a visit to Jeremy Bentham, the utilitarian philosopher. I found him in the cloister of London College sitting in his open wardrobe. Yellow harvest hat, white scarf, black jacket, chestnut pantaloons, white socks and black dancing pumps. He left his body for dissection, but reassembling it to inhabit his clothes was only a partial success. The skeleton was a reasonable fit. But the head and face blacked by sulphuric acid had to be replaced, respectively, by a waxwork and a *trompe l'oeil* mask. His expression resembled the laughing boy in the *Mad Magazine* cartoon.

Bentham used Brunet's concept of the Panopticon to invent a model prison with a tubular design. The resident lord's all-seeing eye was a light at the end of a tunnelled tower, but veiled from the inmates who occupied the exterior, each in solitary confinement, unable to communicate with one another. However, through a pan-optical illusion created by glass-reflections from the tower, each would feel the eye's surveillance every moment of their day and night, and behave themselves accordingly. The idea was squashed by Mad King George who thought he was being mocked by a metaphor. It made Bentham into a utilitarian socialist. His measure of good governance was the greatest happiness of the greatest number. Replace happiness with health, I thought, and you have what Descartes had in mind. The two go together and it's hard to be happy when you're sick.

THE VIRCHOW ENTERPRISE

Before making myself useful I first had to find a trajectory. Two ideas gripped my imagination: Virchow's anthropological law on the interface between medicine and politics, and Bernard Kouchner's *droit d'ingérence*. Kouchner, co-founder of Médecins Sans Frontières, advocated an aggressive form of medical intervention, military if necessary, to rescue exploited peoples sunk in famine and disease. Eliminate the wicked, and the good people will thrive. Kouchner's voice was seductively clear, but it sounded too loud, like a charismatic preacher, drowning out background noise to pound out his message. The thought of a new form of global colonialism based on righteous humanism gave me pause. The solution would be playing the same game of suppression that caused the misery in the first place. I dismissed *ingérence humanitaire* with St Augustine's words, 'Power should be withheld from the righteous.'

Rudolf Virchow (1821-1902) was a celebrated pathologist who went into German politics to oppose Bismarck's empire-building. Unlike Kouchner, his law didn't involve regime change, only a change of heart. 'Medicine is a social science, and politics is nothing but medicine on a larger scale.' His spur was Descartes whose discourse on the centrality of health to the general welfare of mankind had inspired the French Revolution to make medicine a significant arm of the state (arguably for the first time in history). Gentlemen scientists were replaced in the national institutes by vocational biologists, such as Étienne Geoffroy Saint-Hilaire, Georges Cuvier and Jean-Baptiste Lamarck. However, during Bismarck's blinkered reign by blood and iron, Virchow's holistic idea met with deaf ears. He was dismissed as a 'medical mystic', and is only remembered now for his seminal work on the nature of cells.

There was nothing revolutionary about Virchow's basic tenet. The prime object of life is for humans to be as happy and healthy as possible. He was merely prioritising common sense. I decided that while working on the fringes of the established order, I would dedicate myself to asserting his wisdom by indirect action, achieving improvements in the quality of life which would help to invert the primacy of politics over public health. I kept this to myself, as radical ideas like Christianity and Islam are best proven by exemplary enactment.

I was looking for a job where I would be able to get life-enhancing things done in a small way, if possible without being noticed. I would avoid vainglorious ambition, not as a reaction to Mal Combes (he was gloriously vain), but because my child-hood wish to be sight-unseen still prevailed into my middle years. I would quit the mad world of freelance research and find an inconspicuous niche in the mainstream of medicine from which I had hitherto marginalised myself.

My large idea revolved around the gulf between academic research and its application in the real world. This exists since practical implications, not least political consequences, have to be considered. For instance, the hypothesis behind the Good Spit Project and the aborted rice-rat study on tooth loss and ageing was based on Hall McCall's incipient ideas on auto-immunity and Descartes's wistful dream of 'reversing the infirmity of old age'. As the Medical Research Council would have had to con-sider the world historical consequences of ultimately increasing longevity, he obfuscated it when seeking ethical approval and found funding elsewhere.

Macro-solutions require a revolution, and waiting for one in England would be a Spurious Infinity. For example James Douglas's famous cohort studies in the 1940s / 1950s showed that health expectations in the population could only be equalised by the levelling of the class system. Richard Doll and Bradford Hill's studies in the 1950s showing smoking caused cancer and premature births, despite widespread publicity, didn't begin to change habits until almost three decades later when governments, realising its tax potential, invested heavily in health education and price control. By then heart disease and strokes had been added to its undesirable effects. Even so, the tobacco industry, if unable to call the tune any more, could tone it down.

Micro-solutions, incrementally introduced, might help to build up expectations, and be educational without hectoring against what people wanted to do. However, I knew that closing the gap between publication and the application of steady advances can take so long that momentum is lost and the idea is quietly shelved. On the other hand, if the research has a dramatic public profile, and doesn't expect people to change their way of life, the political world jumps to speed it through. For instance, findings on lead in petrol and its damage to children's brains led to its banning before follow-up studies could confirm it. There must be, I thought, unsung breakthroughs lying dormant in the journals, waiting to be implemented. If I identified some feasible examples, I could present myself to Health Authorities with proposals. My mission statement would be, 'Putting Proven Solutions into Practice.'

THE LOW-DOWN ON THE ESTABLISHED ORDER (SEE APPENDIX)

Mal Combes couldn't resist mocking me. 'You are, my poet, thinking like a functionary: achieve the inevitable. And the iron bottoms won't feel challenged.' He was in a roaring good mood because Oswald the guru of Fortnum & Mason's had found Una an eligible Messiah, and they were leaving the cult together. 'The brain-scoop must be furious.' Even when Mal Combes asked me what proven solutions I had in mind, and I had to admit that it was only a notion, and still vague, he praised the idea, saying, 'it will be your point of entry into the inner circle, and in that case you might as well know who's who.' Mal Combes then proceeded to give me a breakdown of the establishment's pecking order. I'll cobble it together from my notes:

The Powers That Be: the politicians with the policies and money bags. Bypass them if you can, but get to know the Opposition MPs. Their pressure can be useful.

The Mandarins: the civil servants who advise the politicians on the consequences of their actions, and tell them how to dole out the money safely. Their clout extends to liaising with local Health Authorities on how the cash is spent. Appeal to their high intelligence. Don't hesitate to call them Mandarins to their face. These inscrutable know-alls are not above ironic flattery. Civil to nobody and servant to the devil is an in-joke. It's said that irony is being amusing about what you don't understand. But with them it's amusement at what they understand only too well.

The Eminent Persons Group: professional advisers to the civil servants. In London I'm the go-between them and the Consultants, who are, of course, God. With them pretend you know more about what's really going on than you do. Try not to mention me. Flatter them. They are not always as sure of themselves as they appear. The ones to watch are Dame Brenda Tabby, Max Madison and Stanley O. Kay. The terrible triumvirate. Brenda, the white Yorkshire rose; Max, the thorn in her side; and Stanley, the buttonhole. You'll be hearing from the Eminents, no doubt.

The Great and Good: the lords and ladies and successful businessmen, who chair committees. They need to be kept sweet if you're to get anywhere. The GGs think they represent the 'real world'. Appeal to their egalitarian vanities. Mention the common weal and they sit up. Suggest the common touch and they stand to attention.

The Health Authorities: the 'self-appointed' bodies who hold the local purse-strings. They are run by executives who know their job, and often have joint posts with the universities. Being accountable to the politicians, and their electorate, they seek advice and listen to it, not least from the Mandarins. Chaired by the Great and Good, they are normally democratic. Exploiting that is useful when trying to influence the less effective authorities.

The Lobby Horses: spokespersons of special interests groups. Sympathise with their cause. Be on their side, no-matter. But if you can't get them on yours, steer them in the direction of the politician most likely to be favourably inclined.

The People Who Matter on the Ground: managers of services. They are for the most part iron bottoms. Some sit, some work. Ability is not a meritocracy. Ask around to find who the doers are. Everybody knows. Either/Or, canvass their advice rhetorically e.g. prepare a plan with apparent prior approval from a higher authority. Sometimes you may need to obfuscate. Above all, be their friend. They feel much put upon.

The Ground Forces: the clinical health workers. A mystical body: all human life is there. Don't expect to understand them as a corporate entity. One thing they have in common. They feel unappreciated. 'We get no support from anyone.'

Be supportive. 'Nobody else is doing their job.' Praise the whiners to the skies. Know that pride in their work reduced by low morale can give them righteous permission to let standards slip. It's why disciplinary proceedings are so high in so-called 'failing' services. Keep your distance. It is possible to offer yourself as a squash partner, or a second violin in their association's orchestra, but never socialise with them. You may have to do things they don't like.

The Upper Echelons: the Consultants. Many in London have private practices on the side. They are in two worlds at the same time. Talk to them and explain that they don't have to do anything. Then make yourself scarce and they will forget you. If you are too obtrusive, you're put in your place. The Royal Colleges and the Medical Council can be invoked. They have the power, but it's no longer absolute. The Mandarins are in confrontation with them. Harness that to progress your ideas if they don't like them. It's a risk worth taking. Keep an ear open for the name their friends and allies call them. It will come in handy when you want to disarm one. If all fails, and some of them want you out, have a word with an old hand like me, or an up-and-coming Consultant. Within the Upper Echelons there are echelons within echelons.

The Underlings: support staff. Don't underestimate what secretaries can do for you behind their bosses' backs. Porters and cleaners are natural spies. The information gained from them in gossip can be invaluable. Know their first names and family history. Share a joke with them.

The Humans: Human Resources are no longer called personnel officers because they advise rather than officiate. Keepers of legal virtue and humane values in the organisation, their priestly and/or psychiatric functions are invaluable. You can talk to them, and even confess your sins or complexes. Choose one, and work solely with her/him.

'In sum, the Mandarins, the Eminent Persons, and the Great and Good maintain the Established Order. The Ground Forces and the Upper Echelons accept this because they have to. The Underlings don't count in the larger scheme of things, but can make the Established Order uncomfortable with their trade unions. In a way, the Health Authorities are outside it. They are supposed to represent the people, and some do.

'The politicians in recent years have become less respectful of the Established Order, and increasingly use managers of service as their Trojan Horses. A new breed from outside the health domain is beginning to replace the iron bottoms. They are less predictable, and can be more flexible when it comes to change. Some will be fools, but they don't tend to last.

'Now you know the cast, and how to play them, the question is who you can trust?'

He handed me a folded page. It was blank. 'Not even my name, Poet. Get one thing right: know that nobody loves anyone else unless they have to.'

Thumbing devil's ears, he concluded, 'Welcome to the portal of hell.'

PAWING THE GROUND

I decided to start with outmoded treatments still in use. Mal Combes was fired up. 'Obsolete materials ordered by Supplies will show them up. Better get the teaching hospitals to identify them. I'll talk to the Dean of Deans, Dean Slowey. It will be a marriage made in heaven: Supplies will save money and the teaching hospitals will save the profession from itself.' He got me an emergency grant from the Mandarins, and I was ready to roll.

The footwork was an unmerry dance. Nobody wanted to give me time. They thought I was a muck-raking journalist. But Mal Combes rang Supplies, and it didn't take long for the troupe of post-graduate students he rounded up to scan the computerised ordering system. A sample list of redundant treatments was presented to the Mandarins, who didn't need to be told that it would be prudent to replace them with proven solutions. At a pub lunch in Soho Mal Combes and a mystery Mandarin made it clear that as far as they were concerned I was the invisible man. I would work quietly with the Ground Forces. Mal Combes said, 'The Eminent Persons Group will want the Consultants to take the lead, and then do nothing.' His final word made the Mandarin smile. 'Consider yourself an experiment, and if it works out, others will follow, even the Eminents. If not, it will be put down to inexperience, and you'll be on a flight to Rio.'

When listed materials or medicines were ordered, I had them stopped. When clinicians complained I went to see them, and explained, offering them the proven alternatives. If they thought I was a rep, and ordered and complained again, I had a standard letter, signed by an appropriate specialist, and myself. Those who had stocked up and didn't need to order were a problem.

I couldn't very well poke around in their cupboards. So I sent them the letter with a request to return unused stock to Supplies, enclosing the original order. If they did nothing or complained to their manager, I paid a visit. These rarely went well. Playing the petty tyrant and laying down the law is no way to parlay. I had to think again.

As I circled around, hell's portal opened on to a quagmire of general unhappiness. Everybody complained about everyone else. At the turn of the 1980s the health service was being broken up into self-managing units called 'trusts'. 'A misnomer,' Mal Combes said. 'Nobody trusts anybody.' Consultants were looking beyond to Harley Street and private work. At least in London and the rich cities. The Ground Forces felt they were in free fall, but carried on as before.

I learned from old-style managers that the sick were getting sicker rather than dying, and monopolising the beds in hospitals, and the well weren't feeling so good and taking up doctors' time. Expansion of services was called for, but contraction was the policy. Clamours for 'new money' were answered with a dull thud. 'There is none. Economies will have to be made,' a euphemism for cuts. 'Existing staff would simply have to work longer hours without overtime pay,' one manager said. 'And that's a Pandora's box nobody wants to open.' Needless to say, the Mandarins had cost-benefit alternatives up their sleeve: cottage hospitals for long-stay patients, and health education clinics for time-wasters and the worried well. But such suggestions were not what the Powers That Be wanted to hear. It was a time for accounting, not ideas.

Indeed, nobody quite knew where the money spent on health was going. The allocation was said to be 'historical', and it was.

The National Health Service was a treasured part of the patrimony, yet it was a stately home described by its architect, Clem Attlee, as 'a house designed by a cat for a dog'. The Beveridge Report, which inspired it, was drafted after a populist war which challenged the class system, and it caught the mood. The language is Miltonic in its metaphors. Five Goliaths were identified for slaying: Idleness, Poverty, Ignorance, Squalor and above all their unfortunate offspring, Sickness.

The country was carried away by David-like feats of legislative reform. It wasn't exactly a 'money no consideration' ethos, but hard cash was secondary to bringing down the giants. The medical profession, largely against it, were lured by financial incentives difficult to refuse rather than Nye Bevan's eloquence. Consultants were offered not only generous terms but independent powers to boot. Retrenchment began in the 1950s, starting with dental and optical charges, but its subsequent execution was opportunist rather than planned with a public health overview.

As a hell it was less Dante's judicious circles than the snakes and ladders of Medici's Florence. Machiavelli would be a more apt guide than the poet's Virgil. I was lucky to have Mal Combes. When my invisibility was impossible to sustain, he changed tack, and spoke on my behalf to the Eminent Persons Group, casually mentioning the Mandarins' support. He was showing solidarity with the Established Order, while betraying what he was doing behind its back. He emphasised that I would report directly to the Eminents, of course, once the project was no longer a departmental experiment. For the unforeseen future I was on my own.

And so the Eminents put in a word on my behalf with the Great and Good, who spoke to the Health Authorities, and after several months pawing the ground, while Mal Combes did the galloping, I found myself entitled to call myself the projects person. The job came with a small budget, and an office that was a converted toilet with the gentlemen sign removed. When I was inside, the latch on the door read 'vacant'. This meant I was not disturbed. Otherwise it was engaged. I had a few complaints about not answering the door, but it added to my mystique. Inaccessibility is the privilege of the invisible.

My office was an improvement on the broom cupboard of my school meals job, and the telephone booths of my Hall McCall-Manders freelance days. It enhanced my feeling that my Virchow enterprise would be undercover, cloak-and-dagger. This excited me. I felt like Dumas's man in the iron mask. Closing my door was like pulling down the visor to make myself anonymous. My contact with the world was notes slipped under my door.

I needed to think. Dealing with outmoded treatments was one thing, introducing new ones would be something else. Outmoders were exceptions. This would be for everybody. The talking in my head was deafening. I knew little about proven solutions. I had to be honest with myself. It was just an idea. But I was ashamed of my ignorance, and it was too late to re-educate myself. Socrates's 'I know that I know nothing' came to my rescue. It was the path of virtue. But the talking in my head taunted me, 'How did Socrates know he knew nothing? Plato doesn't tell us.' I shut it up with Kierkegaard's 'We must learn to know the things we cannot understand'. I wouldn't be taking the hemlock.

I was the ghost in the toilet that no longer worked. I came and went, smiling at those I met in the corridor. I wasn't exactly working covertly. But most people were in the dark as to what I was supposed to be doing. And so was I.

THE BIG IDEA

Mal Combes took me to dinner at the Gay Hussar with its floor-show of tasteful Eastern dancers backed by a slinky sitar. The atmosphere was expensive. The waiters wore livery and you were screened off from other diners by Panopticon ergonomics. The lighting and angle of table placing played their part.

'So you're a projectionist at last, Poet. You always wanted to work in the dark. What's your programme?'

'I'm still in the process of clarifying who my audience is.'

'Your audience? I don't see anyone queuing outside your privy.'

'In the cinema of life the audience is always a loner.'

'So you're your own audience?'

'No. Thanks to you I will be reporting directly to the Eminents.'

'So you'll always be on your own.'

But our verbal floats and speech melodies were not in accord with the sitar's dervish dance. Mal Combes wanted to know what I was going to do next and I hadn't an idea.

'And so, my Jack of All Trades, you're a servant, more or less, of what I come up with.' He guffawed rather too loudly for my liking.

'You never laugh at your own jokes, Master. Ergo, it's no joke.' I mimicked Nasty's mocking tone.

'Spit it out, Poet. What's your big idea? I'm all ears.'

I trusted Mal Combes. Not many would. We both knew he would double-cross me if he had to, but he would make up for it in other ways. Above all I trusted him not to laugh at my ideas. He was the only person that I didn't mind calling me a poet. So I verbally floated a vague plan.

'Apart from being old stagers, most of the outmoders worked on their own. They felt they were being singled out, and took it badly. Either they abased themselves horribly or stood their ground like mongooses. This is time-consuming, and rather miserable, and augurs ill for putting proven solutions into practice. And so I'm thinking about an open forum with groups of colleagues from different generations. Pascal says that people are best persuaded by what they come by themselves.'

'Peer review,' said Mal Combes. 'It's routine in any self-respecting hospital.'

'I don't have any new ideas, only old ones given a new life.'

'Dean Slowey will jump at the chance to try out peer review in the real world.'

He put a ten pound note in the belly dancer's girdle, and said, 'Get your idea clear and after that you can distort it as you please.' His wink to the dervish was acknowledged with an offhand nod.

It was to be my last free meal out with Mal Combes. Perhaps he no longer considered me a student. Or he didn't want to be seen with me alone. Or now that Una was off his hands, he didn't need me for anything beyond the call of duty. Still, maybe there is no great mystery about it. Some things happen, or do not, without a larger plan.

FIRST STEPS

Without telling Mal Combes, I made an appointment with Dean Slowey, and outlined my little big idea. I had rustled up a few examples of proven solutions. Nothing earthshaking. They sounded hardly worth mentioning. As he said nothing,

I had no speech melodies to go by, and verbal-floated on about herbal remedies that Hervě Thuau, my medical anthropologist, swore by. I thought I'd blown it when I ambled into an account of a pandemic study of zinc peroxide in tissue repair in Maoist China. Its effectiveness was tested on all cases of traffic accidents occurring during a week (I'd heard about it in a documentary film on the Red Guard's Cultural Revolution at the Anarchist Society in the Drill Hall).

Dean Slowey finally spoke. 'I like the idea. Leave the rest to the experts. Most of my departments will be only too pleased to make suggestions. You can count on that. Come back when you have a concrete proposal.' I almost burst into tears.

Realising I had forgotten to mention the supporting peer review idea, I made another appointment with his secretary on the way out, and the next day I found myself recounting my experiences with the outmoders over lunch with the Dean. He asked me for the list of redundant treatments. I rolled them off as though I was an expert. 'O yes, I remember them well,' was his amused reaction.

Emboldened, I enlarged the picture by confiding to him Edna Gray's work in the Reimbursement Board. I had kept in contact with her and she was well on the way to establishing a democracy of good practice: measuring the average distribution of clinical activities weighted for the particular population. I said that computerisation of treatment payments offered the most unobtrusive way of identifying atypical performances, and possible malpractice. For instance, doctors with an unusually high patient death-rate could be picked out for further investigation. Dean Slowey's eyebrows twitched.

Excitedly, I added that Edna Gray's index could in theory be applied to all clinicians in the peer review groups as a control.

Their itemised payments are with Edna Gray. Dean Slowey interrupted me. 'It would be illegal. I understand Edna's remit is to find methods to detect fraud. The Medical Council would want to know if she went beyond that. It has shock-horror implications: computer surveillance of every practitioner in the land. No government would dare…'

In the heat of the moment, I had forgotten it was a secret, and immediately reassured him that it was merely for Edna's own personal use. 'Trust Edna,' he laughed. 'She thinks national statistics are her own private property.' He relaxed, and talked about her. They had been to college together in Durham, and were friends. 'But, for goodness sake, don't mention to a soul her tinkering with data. Edna gets carried away by ideas. And this one is no less brilliantly dangerous than usual.'

Buoyed up by Dean Slowey, I was ready to enter unknown territories. A surge of Leibniz's *optimisme* drowned out the talking in my head. I would bring Virchow's idea into practice by the back door until it was recognised as a world view. My sense of getting away with things was to the fore, not as a fear of being found out, but as a feeling of impending triumph. One day, maybe not in my lifetime, the politics of medicine would become the medicine of politics, and my closet machinations might well have contributed to it in a small way. But the talking in my head resurfaced. It was a struggle not to embarrass myself when I entertained larger ideas.

THE SUPPLICANT

Existential embarrassment was not an issue with Mal Combes. He might embarrass me, but not himself. That he shamelessly used people did not bother me. My ambitions were cosmic rather than personal, and Virchow had an inadvertent champion in him. His manipulations of the Established Order could be said to tally with the attacks from within that usually precede revolutions.

No matter what he did, or didn't do, I could not take against Mal Combes. He saw me for what I was worth to him, but, if I failed to deliver the goods, he didn't reproach me. There was always a next time. Despite two-timing him with Dean the Dean Slowey, he was talking about me in the right places. And when I got an appointment to speak at a Great and Good seminar, I didn't need to ring him up to thank him.

As I would only have five minutes I changed my mission statement into a strap-line: 'Making what is supposed to happen happen.' Virchow's idea was somewhere in there, but reduced to an action rather than a crusade. The Great and Good didn't like the implied criticism of the health services coming from anyone except themselves.

Lord Peter, a Labour peer, questioned whether, inadvertently or not, there could be a conflict of interest or, even, a vested interest, say, the drug companies, and whether this could compromise my project. Ivor Bell-Smith, a new boy amongst the Great and Good, pointed out that effectively I was putting myself forward as a troubleshooter and only the government had the right to appoint one. On the other hand, Lady Wilton liked the corporateness of peer review. 'Everybody together.' I didn't tell her I got the idea from my days as an anarchist: the group decides. However, the Great and Good were not dismissing my ideas. They suggested I put together a position paper with the Eminents for them to present to the Health Authorities.

I shuddered. If my project became a matter of paper, even if I got the go-ahead, the Eminents would fire the shots and my ammunition would be blanks. I told them it was an experiment, and the results would be a departmental matter. They were not best pleased. The Chair said, 'it is a matter of public interest, not security,' and spoke at length on the importance of transparency and the common weal, and keeping in touch with the public. He spoke to me as to the nation, and it was made clear my place was as a supplicant in the inner sanctum.

The balance of power it seemed was not much different from that of the nineteenth century. De Tocqueville's view that 'governance in England is by rule of club not by rule of mob' still held strong. The Established Order was self-sustaining. Or was it? Rumour had it that the mob was gathering at the gate. But who or what were they storming? The Mandarins were encouraging their ministers to bypass the Great and Good, and work more closely with the Eminents. I was an emissary from the Mandarins, suspected of being barricade material, posing as a lackey of the Established Order. Their confidence in me, albeit guarded, came with the supercilious indulgence afforded an idealist with a worthy, but impractical, idea. It could be read as a sign of weakness. I felt a suspicion of embarrassment on their behalf as though I were an outsider who had entered the stadium without a ticket, and been given a seat next to executives of the losing side.

As nothing much was happening, I used the pause to get out more to make my presence felt. I was no longer the invisible man. I organised my rounds to coincide with the People That Mattered coming out of important meetings. A verbal float with a Great and Good, or even a passing politician was well received and noticed by others. I gave the impression of knowing every-body when, in fact, I was chancing my arm with people who had only seen me maybe once or twice. I pretended to be on familiar terms with them. Mal Combes's advice on putting names to faces came in handy.

Each of his categories had to be approached differently. I became all things to all men, preparing my verbal floats down to the last pleasantry. When their speech melodies didn't sing, I passed on with a friendly touch on the shoulder and a part-ing float (mystique retained). I took risks, exposing myself to more chance encounters, appearing as people were breaking for lunch or going home. I diversified into secretaries and cleaners. It involved improvisation, as responses were not predictable. I remembered what Nasty said about my declining capacity to think on my feet, and took it as a challenge. When the ground began to move under me I needed to learn how to move with it.

DUMMY RUN

Dean Slowey wrote the position paper for me, more or less. He was nearing retirement and 'wanted to go out with a flourish,' he said. 'I've passed most of my adult life within the confines of academia, and missed out on the real world.' It wasn't just about retraining doctors and dentists. He saw the potential of outreach clinics for research and development, and teaching hospital ratings were based on that. He replaced 'peer review' ('too military') with 'clinical audit', saying, 'audit is the man-na-word of the moment.' He didn't use magic. And so I guessed that he had been reading Roland Barthes, and said so. 'Yes, the mystery word that gives the impression of being the answer to everything.'

'Like "the flesh of the world".'

'Ah, Merleau-Ponty. I'm catching up belatedly with "the incarnation of the mind". If the body does the thinking, not consciousness, there is hope for us all.'

'Then he spoils it all by saying, "The perceiving mind cannot be disentangled from the perceived". That's Bishop Berkeley in a solipsist's hell.'

'I'm not sure I understand you.'

'Neither am I.'

But Dean dug out a design of Jeremy Bentham's Panopticon prison from a book on his library shelf. And together we worked it out in Berkeleyan terms, *To be is to be perceived.*

'It's a game of hide and seek,' I said.

'Seek and you will find. Knock and the door will open.'

And in came his secretary.

We had the kind of conversations that Dr Thrower (Up) craved for, perhaps. Only Dean Slowey's universe was a benign one. He had Michel Foucault's *Birth of the Clinic* on his desk. I said I got stuck reading it. 'It's the translation,' he said. 'One day I'll read it in French.' But we both had it in for Foucault for his subjugation of the subjective self to the supposed objective reality. 'He's an extremist of self-effacement,' Dean sighed, 'and at the same time cloyingly arrogant.' That rang a bell.

The Eminents detected Dean Slowey's master hand in the position paper, and promptly passed it on to the Department of Health with their seal of approval. And the rest was plain sailing. The peer review was given the go as a pilot project. Service managers who wanted to be ahead of prescriptive planning were eager to try it out. I didn't want to dampen down their enthusiasm by telling them to wait till the new academic year for the specialist placements. But I wasn't doing much, and at Dean Slowey's departments I updated myself on topics for clinical audit that I already knew something about, such as cross-infection control. A dummy run would be in order. Afternoon sessions were organised for the groups to audit their clinical practices.

My sessions started nervously. Nobody wants to change the way they work. Firm conclusions were resisted. However, once the groups relaxed, clinicians welcomed the sharing, even expressing relief at being able to talk openly about their own methods. A certain cordiality emerged between the generations. Amusement at what the older clinicians were taught was tempered by awe at the placebo effect. At first I kept minutes of the agreed protocol. But since the participants themselves were establishing the consensus, I withdrew after my preamble and, providing secretarial assistance, left them to be their own amanuensis.

As I gained confidence, when a recalcitrant Peer Group was getting nowhere, and what was supposed to happen didn't, I willed an embarrassing scene. When comparisons with other groups did not shame them, I gave up gentle persuasion and became deliberately rude ('Now listen to me. I've heard all that before. You're like dogs chasing their own tails.'). A blunt statement with no suggestion of sarcasm worked to clear the air, and often united them to prove me wrong. However, when embarrassing them by losing my patience, I found I embarrassed myself. And next session I apologised to everyone and was especially nice. But eating humble pie reversed the transference. Everyone was embarrassed.

Sometimes that brought us together but, more often than not, I remained the enemy, and played the part. Fired up, I would see how far I could go, bombarding them with desperate exaggerations designed to get to the bottom of their sincere objections. Throwing a scene I knew could go horribly wrong. I tried to make it more like barn-storming theatre, sometimes shamelessly stage Irish. My hope was it would end in laughter, and some progress would be possible. If it ended in tears and complaints, I could explain to their manager that it was just group role play (bringing out the existential embarrassment in others to unburden one's own. A human move Ian Russell introduced me to).

TESTING TIMES

I was testing people, I suppose, like Jack Black, the Aids activist and ex-African missionary. He was a broth of a boy with five brothers, all over six foot five, back on the family farm in Co. Meath. That he was two inches shorter could have accounted for the lengths he went to prove himself in the fight for the acceptance of Aids as a normal disease in the mid-eighties. He led marches with the banner 'I am HIV positive', and became the most prominent carrier in London. He used to cut a finger and present himself with a friend at casualty in hospitals, and shake hands with doctors and nurses (who knew him well) to see if they would flinch at the seeping bandage. And if they did so he had them on film – his friend carried a hidden camera. He spoke directly to it, stating dried blood could not carry the virus, as they ought to know, and that their reaction was a primitive prejudice against people living with HIV. It never made the evening news but was widely circulated. I included it in peer review sessions on cross-infection control.

Jack Black was the longest HIV carrier of first generation positives. 'Only the prostitutes of Gabon could compete with me,' he boasted. So powerful was Jack Black that when he headed a protest march, it was said the police horses hesitated. His dentist broke a bone on his little finger trying to extract a molar buried in his lantern jaw. The anaesthetic injection was not working properly but Jack Black did not wince, and the dentist ended up in casualty with Jack Black holding his hand. People wondered how he caught HIV. As an ex-Gaelic football player it had to be women. When he began to appear everywhere with a handsome Brazilian with a ring in his ear it did the world of good for the image of homosexuals. He was testing prevailing prejudices. Later he was seen pushing a pram full of black-and-white babies. I wanted to shake hands with him for widening the game, but there was a crowd around him. Everybody loved Jack Black.

NEEDLES IN THE BUSHES

Upon the advent of Dean Slowey's specialists, my role as actor-manager was mercifully curtailed. They were teachers and knew how to perform (and behave). The peer review was rapidly subsumed into the system, and ceased to be a pilot. I would have to think of something else to do. I got the usual phone call: 'I want you to do something for me, Poet.' I said yes before I knew what it was.

Chiropodists and dentists were refusing to treat HIV carriers. As the foot and mouth were often focuses of opportunist infections with Aids patients, Mal Combes had in mind a dedicated clinic in St Margaret's Hospital near where the main Aids charity was located. I would be expected to find staff and get the service started. 'How's the money?' I asked, and he laughed. 'Money for Aids isn't a problem. Spending it is because there is no known cure. It's no secret the pot of gold is being pilfered from by everybody.'

Jack Black put me in touch with gay dentists and chiropodists who were only too keen to man the foot-and-tooth clinic evenings and weekends. Refurbishing the suite and equipping it was made easy by them. And it was up and running in record time. However, when hospital staff saw all these pale, interesting young men in the waiting room, they began to talk. At that time most HIV carriers were homosexuals, and two sets of prejudices became confused with each other. Hospital patients and the families joined in with complaints, and the hospital manager banished the service to Portakabins in the grounds, where porters refused to collect mail or rubbish. They would deliver only.

Aids charities were up in arms. When a black bag of contaminated waste was found strewn in the bushes the service was closed down. It was said the bag had been planted as a protest by the HIV lobby. I checked the items and the waste tallied with that of a surgical theatre rather than a foot-and-tooth clinic. Clearly a homophobic nurse or doctor had dumped it there. But nobody listened to me. However, a former brothel in Victoria was found to rehouse the clinic, and everybody was happy.

Jack Black was fomenting direct action in Peterborough. A man had been found slumped in his car after an assault. He was taken to the hospital, where doctors tested his blood and found that he was infected with HIV. Environmental health officials were called out and the street was cordoned off while council workers in protective clothing fumigated the area. Traffic was diverted for two days while the toxic disinfectant evaporated. When the pound refused to tow the car away, an Aids charity arranged to find its rightful home. The police provided a cortège of motorcycles. The man's name was not revealed, presumably to save his family the shame. Subsequently he was found to be a registered drug addict. Aids wasn't just the gay plague. Jack Black marched through the city with a giant needle. The placard read, 'Knitting causes Aids'. Fun and games.

Meanwhile, I hadn't quite escaped from peer review. Dean Slowey contacted me to ask what should be done with certain clinicians within it who were clearly not up to their job. 'Some are a serious danger to patients,' he said. I suggested that we apply Edna Gray's index to them. Then pass the result on to their professional bodies. I wasn't joking. But Dean seemed amused…

I knew who they were. Endless complaints about them had come my way, ranging from alcohol on the breath to sheer bloody-mindedness. Burnout was putting it kindly. I spoke to Human Resources, and retraining as usual was recommended. But it had already been tried by the respective trust managers. Even peer review, a form of retraining with collective responsibility to the fore, had failed to move them. Their burnout was ashes to dust from which no phoenix was likely to rise. Recourse to employment law would be necessary.

And so I took a crash course in disciplinary procedures with Cassandra O'Flynn, an Irish girl with no side, and a mind of her own. Engaging with the intricacies of the process, I realised a law without a Hegelian escape clause had caught up with my pragmatism. The sod-it get-out to end hesitations could not be applied. Spurious Infinities beckoned.

The talking in my head was silent and the writing on the wall blank. I felt my life would never be the same. Perhaps I needed to revisit my autochthonous indwellers, the onlie begetters of the earliest written law in Western Europe, circa fourth century. Inscribed on stone pillars in Ogham was an alphabet taking its twenty-five letters from the names of trees. Maybe they knew the wood from...

IV

WHAT THE AUTOCHTHONES IN MY BLOOD TOLD ME

'The old people in my blood I honour with a sigh.'

—E. M. Cioran

SHAKESPEARE'S IRISH?

MY OLD PEOPLE CAME TO ME THROUGH GAELIC poetry, and I sighed at my lingering ambition to honour them. I had only ever written poems in English. Gaelic, my other language, was all but dead. Yet, as I had not lost my accent, it remained Oirish-English. Neither had I lost my Irish accent in metrical matters. I had inherited from my father's teacher, Austin Clarke, his prosodic ideas on the influence of the Gaelic Bardic School on Irish-English verse. I avoided metre, the regular heartbeat of English poetry, and went for the fibrillations of syllabic verse. Rhyme was its crowning topping and tailing, I opined. But Ian Russell disagreed: 'A rhyme cannot be true to English ears unless you have the received pronunciation. The BBC has standardised it.' True enough, but who else spoke it?

Shakespeare's sonnets are usually taken as the model of what poetry in vernacular English should be. Scholars at Joab Comfort's university at that time had been examining his rhymes to divine how the Bard of Avon spoke. Joab played me a recording, and it was clear from the elided rhymes that Shakespeare talked with a pronounced brogue ('agin' for again, 'pin' for pen, 'tay' for tea). Stratford-upon-Avon is closer to Wales than London, and Wales is halfway to Ireland.

We then moved on to studying the verbal floats of Captain Macmorris, the only Irishman in Shakespeare's plays. He is afforded a scattering of 226 words in *Henry V*. Macmorris is an officer of the King's army on the retreat. Insinuations that he is a treacherous Irishman rouse his ire. Mimicking Shakespeare's brogue, I spoke his interjections. But the bad spelling and worse grammar made him seem a comic outsider rather than a hardened warrior. And so I melded his snippets into a single speech, and respecting Shakespeare's "ishes' and 'tises', recited it, chug-lipped:

> By Chrish, la, tish ill-done! The work ish give over. The town is beseech'd... and the trompet call us to the breach; and we talk, and, be Chrish, do nothing. 'Tis shame for us all, so God sa' me, 'tis shame to stand still; it is shame, by my hand; and there is throats to be cut and work to be done... What is my nation? Ish a villain, and a bastard, and a knave, and a rascal. What ish my nation? Who talks about my nation... I do not know you so good a man as myself. So Chrish save me, I will cut off your head.

'Spoken like a true Corkman,' Joab said. Shakespeare must have overheard the rump of Shane ('The Proud') O'Neill's entourage when the last of the fiery Irish chieftains made his ill-judged submission to Queen Elizabeth. Shane's disintegrating train of soldiers and entertainers were stranded in London. Elizabeth had detained him beyond his resources ('English diplomacy at its usual game,' Joab said), and his bards went a-begging in the streets, and stayed because there was nowhere else to go. They could well have been joined by gleemen from Munster when their traitor chieftain, the Earl of Ormonde, bent the knee to Elizabeth by becoming a Protestant. Later in the play Shakespeare has the Cockney Pistol misquote a Waterford song, 'Cailín ó cois tSuire mé' ('A girl from beside the River Suir am I') in mockery of his French prisoner's protestations:

> 'Je suis le gentilhomme de bonne qualité.'
> 'Cality! Calen o custure me.'

The 'fighting Irish' find it difficult to make themselves understood without violence, but their sweet songs live on. I continued writing occasional verse in my own brogue after consulting my autochthonous indwellers, and Joab Comfort. According to him 'the arboreal alphabet of Ogham is a MacGuffin. The writing on the stone pillars pertains to property rights, not anything poetical.' Nevertheless, since 'Trespassers will be prosecuted' was translated by Dante into his vernacular as 'Lasciate ogni speranza, voi ch'entrate' ('Abandon all hope, ye who enter here'), I said, 'hell, sod-it,' and made an Ogham poem on midway through life waking up in a dark forest.

MY SECRET WEAPON

When I first came to London and was looking for digs I came across a 'No blacks or Irish' notice in Dagenham. I went in, and presented my reference letter as I thought one should. The landlady led me to a room, calling me 'doctor'. It would have done me fine but I thanked her and said, 'No. It's only fit for blacks or Irish.' She burst into tears.

Two decades later, being Irish had become more acceptable, largely due to the second generation of emigrants making their mark. Indeed, Irishness was only openly scoffed at by their parents. But I remained self-conscious about my origins. Sometimes I wondered was I making too much of them in cosmopolitan London? Jack Black wore his proudly on his sleeve and nobody seemed to mind. Irishry had advanced sufficiently in literary circles to be ironised by Anthony Powell in his journals. 'The Irish man, like the homosexual, has an eternal subject of conversation.' But, although things had changed since my Dagenham days, I thought the more things change on the surface, the more they stay the same in the subconscious.

As a freelancer, when my Irishness was remarked upon, I had a standard response: '*Integendeel*, I'm Dutch.' My Lowland '*au contraire*' shut them up. But, once I had a job with some status, my nationality was a moot subject. Nobody mentioned it, except me. Then only as a last resort, as with the peer review recalcitrants. Still I knew it was observed, and no doubt used to explain unusual aspects of my comportment when people were talking amongst themselves. My verbal floats and bouts of extreme bluntness were cause for ethnic comment.

I was not displeased with my position. What could be seen as a disadvantage was an asset. I could use my Irishness, and English colleagues couldn't, at least directly. I did not disguise my accent, but spoke very distinctly (like my mother on the phone). I decided it was a magical weapon like Fionn MacCool's *gae-bolg* (spear). It entered the enemy like a javelin and its barbs opened up inside. By slipping in the odd begorrah or bejasus, I sometimes tempted them into an indiscretion – for instance, an Irish joke. I didn't respond to it myself, but watched to see if someone else would take them to task. I had nothing to lose, and could gain the moral high ground by default. It was a useful version of transference in embarrassment.

Once Max Madison of the Eminents tittered something about the Queen's English at my deliberate 'muddling' of Reginald Maudling's name (as Secretary of State for Northern Ireland, Maudling was openly contemptuous of Irish people). I pretended I did not hear Max, and my very English reaction was appreciated by others present. 'Silence seduces the truth' (René Char) in more ways than one. The unpleasantness passed.

Irishness gave me a left-handed form of power. Freedom to slip in and out of the mainstream at will. My mother had told me that the Englishman knows his place and the place of others. That held for fellow natives. But the place of a professional Irishman who didn't try to integrate was ambiguous. I was neither a timeserver, nor the enemy within, and certainly not 'one of us'. This made the Great and Good uneasy. I was to be considered a maverick, which meant I was allowed to get away with outrageous remarks. 'A breath of fresh air,' warbled Lady Wilton. But on balance I don't think she liked draughts. As many of the Mandarins were Scottish, my Irishness was taken for granted. But the Eminents were something else. Not taking me seriously was their mode of discourse.

'He's a bit of a card,' Stanley O. Kay, their chairperson said. 'An *enthusiast*.' That pulled me up. It suggested hyperactive sebaceous glands and bad body odour. But Hemingway's 'sweating off the fat of civilisation' was a phrase that the latent anarchist in me approved of, and I relaxed with it, not unhappy to be placed in the bathhouse of those who were trying to clean me up, in order to be made presentable. 'Fat chance of that,' the talking in my head said. I basked in the thought that I could never be dressed up to be part of the Established Order. On its outer skin I would be a rubefacient, a useful irritant.

'I've learned how to rock the boat without getting into it,' I boasted to Ian Russell at one of our Sunday evenings. But, the appellation *enthusiast* still rankled. I shared Voltaire's definition of it with Ian: 'Enthusiasm is not always the companion of total ignorance. It is more than often the result of erroneous information.'

'You will have to be more assiduous in checking your sources then,' he said. 'On the other hand, Voltaire claimed that there was a nerve between the mouth and the heart in humans, turtledoves and pigeons, which is why they are the only animals that kiss.'

'Maybe there is merit in chancing my arm, or imagination.'

'That's what poetry is for.'

So we improvised a duet:

> 'You don't take yourself seriously enough.'
> 'For that, my too-kind friend, I'd need self-love.
> I've never been serious in my own eyes.'
> 'Leave it to others.' 'That would be a surprise.'

'WHAT IS MY NATION?' (*Shakespeare*)

Like Captain Macmorris, the Irishman in Shakespeare's plays, I never thought of England as my country. I was too interested in the natives' reaction to mine, and to me as a foreigner. My commitment to England was a matter of industry rather than identification. There were works to be done, if not throats to be cut. On the other hand, I no longer lived in Ireland, except in dreams, and short holidays to see my mother. Before I left, family expectations on my behalf were low. But I refused my place as the fool of the family. Heredity be damned. I had to believe I sprang from my own loins. I would gird them myself. Descartes had given me a lifeline, and Virchow an idea that I wanted to bring to life. A forlorn hope, perhaps, but one with an object. I would live it.

I saw George Bernard Shaw's *John Bull's Other Island* in Malvern, a town which for me exemplified Englishness at its most paramount. It was the year of the Malvinas adventure, a fleet sent to the South Atlantic to save an outpost of Little England. The play wasn't taken as a comedy by the matinee audience, but as a moral betrayal, a treason. They almost hissed at the actor playing Broadbent, (rather too broadly, I thought). Englishmen that were more Irish than the Irish themselves were known to me. They had the ridiculousness of the converted, and stood out like sore thumbs. Holding their pints higher than everybody else, these back-thumpers peppered their brogue with Gaelic jabberwocky. I exaggerate, but so did they.

I wasn't invited to public dinners, or dinner parties, but I had a pass into the inside track as the designated scapegoat. If anyone in authority needed a foil or a fool I was available. My niche was uncertain enough to be inhabited without feeling I belonged to anyone or anywhere. It perched me on a prop in the wings, looking laterally on to the theatre of influence, ever alert to the noises off. 'Our Irish friend is of course politically naïve,' I overheard Dame Brenda Tabby pronounce. My confidence grew every time I heard something I wasn't supposed to. I was a Trojan Horse on my own behalf.

Knowing that the politically-naïve *enthusiast* was not considered a threat made me less of a lamb to slaughter. I began to pride myself as having side, but no back. The knife would, I thought, slide off me. But the Eminents were not my only enemy. Apart from myself, there were the recalcitrants and errant clinicians, and possibly people I didn't know. But if I didn't get my retaliation in first, there would always be Mal Combes to pick me up, and find me something to do, or maybe I could go to America where I had a cousin who was Rockefeller's housekeeper.

Becoming English in any way was unthinkable. My revolutionary father would have turned in his grave. Although, after the War of Independence, he and his brother (who robbed guns from the Chelsea Barracks and stood trial during the Anglo-Irish Treaty negotiations in 1921) rented a car and made a pilgrimage around the Cathedral towns of England, and so lingering bad feelings were lessened. But my mother said that my father loved English culture but never trusted the English. He had been part of the Irish delegation officially as an advisor on Northern Ireland, but really to find out what Lloyd George was saying to his private secretary in Welsh ('They were merely exchanging pleasantries'). However, he overheard Churchill joking to Lord Birkenhead, 'The Ulster Unionists needn't worry. What Collins has signed will divide his own side. And what David has signed will divide Ireland.'

Yet in London I didn't feel I was living with the enemy. The English were almost outnumbered by the foreigners. And things had moved on. Post-Beveridge, England had full employment and a need for immigrants. Above all, it had an all-inclusive welfare state paid for by tax. At its inception Nye Bevan, faced by the British Medical Council's opposition to a National Health Service (doctors, used to lucrative private practice, didn't want to part with patients' money), successfully wooed Conservative Party support. Bevan told them, 'We ought to be proud, despite our financial and economic anxieties, that we are able to do the most civilised thing in the world: put the welfare of sick people before any other consideration.' If Virchow is feasible anywhere it is here, I told myself, shyly.

Moreover, there was no question of it working in Ireland, where mother and child state support had been outlawed by the Church because it interfered with the family. I had recently been invited to apply for a job in the university department that I had left in virtual disgrace, and declined. I was only asked because O'Hickee recommended me, and I doubted Virchow would hold holy water there.

BLOOD

I received an invitation to the Queen's Garden Party. It wasn't by divine right, but a lucky dip for healthcare workers. The card lacked gold borders and the royal seal. The only inscription was in French, RSVP. Not having the clothes, I tore it up, and regretted it immediately. I had missed a chance to see how 'the people in-between' behaved in the presence of royalty. And maybe just as well. Security clearance would have opened a Pandora's box, if the officials could have read my mind.

A few years earlier, I had an appointment with ambiguity but I didn't realise it. Escaping from the laboratory on a wet afternoon, I went to the movies. The Odeon picture palace was already crumbling into a bingo hall. At the box office a claw-like hand passed me a ticket. I made out a few slumped forms in the dim-lit auditorium.

I had no idea what was showing. Chance threw me a reissue of *The Reckoning* in which Nicol Williamson is a top business-man who, on returning to Liverpool for his father's funeral, learns belatedly the death was due to a bar fight. Teddy boys taunted his father because of his Irish accent and it turned nasty. Rediscovering his Irish roots, Williamson's blood is up and he vows to wreak vengeance.

Hunger strikes had just started in Northern Ireland, an extreme event that no Irishman could think about without a historical shudder (While Brehon Law made fasting a means of obtaining justice, and Catholicism made it a virtue, the Great Famine aligned it with persecution, and it became a lethal instrument of passive violence). I struggled to be even-handed. I was angry with the British government and the IRA, and ashamed at the same time (Milton's ambiguity, 'A double sense of deluding'). And so I had transcribed a passage of AE (George Russell) as a warning to myself not to go tribal, and pinned it to my noticeboard:

In the shadows in Ireland, North and South, lurks reptilian human life, bigots who in the name of Christ spit on His precepts, and who have put on the whole armoury of hate. Men, and women too, who have known the dark intoxication of blood, and who seek half-consciously for the renewal of that sinister ecstasy.

(*Irish Homestead*, 1922)

But to no avail. In the dark of a flea-pit watching a good bad movie my blood was up. Starving yourself to death in order to be recognised as a political prisoner blasphemed against their religion (suicide is the only unforgivable sin), and against nature (we're all big hungry boys). But it's the ritual redemption of Irish republican despair. It didn't merit the ghoulish ignorance of the tabloid press with its cheap gibes, and the supercilious indifference of English politicians, apart from Red Ken Livingstone. Attempts to force-feed these young men failed.

I thought of Terence MacSwiney, the Lord Mayor of Cork, who made a one-man famine of himself after the Black and Tans burnt down his city. MacSwiney was, by all accounts, a gentle, intelligent man, more a hunger-artist than a rebel. He was his own lost cause. Before the 1916 Rising Patrick Pearse had proclaimed, 'Life springs from death and from the graves of patriots spring living nations,' recalling a sticker that I had recently spotted on a litterbin in Kilburn: 'Honour Ireland Dead [*sic*]'. I left the cinema with the dark intoxication boiling in my blood, certain of one thing. I was in enemy territory, and the only weapon I had was to put my body on the line. Only when I hit the frail tenuous light of the high street did I come to my senses. I remembered MacSwiney's widow's remark, 'Every English person I come across is killable. I regard them as a plague of moral lepers,' and squirmed.

Tower Hamlets may be black and white on a dull day, but life is not. The rush of blood to my brain drained to my feet. I wanted to run like I did as a boy when I wished I was someone else. But it would only attract attention to me. I asked myself how was I capable of reacting with such violence to so slight a film? The plot was *Hamlet,* the avenging of a murdered father. But Nicol Williamson, the prince, certainly didn't hesitate in hunting down the teddy boys. The plot was stock B-movie with an unconvincing racist twist (in Liverpool at the time an Irish accent would not be cause for comment). Above all, the degeneration of Williamson's dulcet English tones into the demonic brogue Marlon Brando used in *The Nightcomers* was laughable. *Darby O'Gill and the Little People* came to mind. I was myself again. The writing was on the screen.

And so the 'big' dropped out of my ambiguities, and I was left with 'amities', sitting in a pub listening to two women in an adjacent cubicle. Their backs were to me. But I could guess from the heavy coats and scarves, and cosily relaxed mien, that they were two old friends enjoying an afternoon drink.

'I want his body for a half an hour.'

'What do you want it for?'

'Never mind. It's none of your business.'

'Remember that little girl.'

'I want that body.'

'I know what you mean.'

They didn't look like body or baby snatchers. And the voices were not lowered as though they were sex-abusers exchanging confidences. I was too polite to strain to get a better look. I wondered if I'd heard them right, and glued my ear to every word. But they had moved on to talk about dressmaking. I finished my coffee and left, none the wiser. So much for the body.

My mind's security clearance might also have led to detention for contemplated regicide. Years back, an outbreak of foot-and-mouth disease prevented me going home to Ireland to see my mother. On Christmas Day I drove to Windsor on empty roads to give myself a breath of fresh air in the grounds of the castle. As I passed the chapel a party poured out – tall seedy-looking men in suits, their handsome horsey consorts, and a little old lady in her Sunday best. The Queen and I were close enough to touch. There were a few people in the courtyard watching with mild interest, thinking no doubt the royal family look better on television. I was wearing an orange oilskin, under which I could have had the shotgun my father used against the Black and Tans.

My chances of getting away with a pot-shot were good, I surmised. Not a policeman in sight. The only time I ever contemplated an act of violence was by proxy at a film (what happened on the rugby field was unpremeditated). I was Godard's existential anti-hero in *Pierrot le Fou* swinging into a gratuitous act with a bomb planted in a golf ball. And, indeed, the sudden appearance of the royal family was as unreal as a New Wave movie being shot. The door on the set was open, and anything could walk in. And I was anything, the intruder, wielding a conceptual weapon. However, other than the Queen's symbolic significance, I had nothing against this woman, who looked indeed like everybody else's mother, and was trying to make herself agreeable with a little yellow smile and a flutter of the wrist. I couldn't help waving back as the royal family disappeared into a side building.

Cheered, I recited to myself Prospero's 'Our revels now are ended. These our actors, as I foretold you, were all spirits and are melted into thin air...' But the gorgeous palaces and unsubstantial pageants didn't quite fade. Even if my imaginary gun had materialised into the real thing and the precept to act came to me and I shot her point-blank, it wouldn't make any difference. One of the dandruffy men with bad complexions would be crowned king. The symbol would live on, a mirage of an analogy which allowed English people to escape from the present on ceremonial occasions.

But the absence of media cameras indicated that royalty was losing its bowing power. The House of Windsor was to languish as a joke, or an outrageous expense, until a wayward princess with a kind heart in the latter decades of the twentieth century, resuscitated the royalty as reluctant celebrities. I was to watch Lady Di's funeral cortège stopping traffic under the flyover at Hendon. Thousands of people were looking down in a deadly silence unheard of in London.

A decade after the spurned Garden Party, I bumped into Princess Anne by accident. The defunct Samaritan Hospital in Soho had been converted into an all-purpose community centre. The manager crashed his car speeding to attend the inauguration. I came to make up for the missed Garden Party, arriving on my bike at the last minute. The Princess was waiting in the lobby with the Great and Good, and local politicians. It was hastily decided that those involved in the planning would do the honours and conduct her around. I had set up a minor surgery clinic for training doctors and dentists, and contributed to a poly-care facility for homeless people. Both were on the first floor, and so the royal party was waiting for me.

I removed my bicycle clips and borrowed a tie (grey to match my purple shirt and white slacks. Cyclists need to be seen), and shaking her delicate hand, I apologised for being late. I was caught in the traffic. Graciously she said, 'I should apologise to you. It was my lot that caused the jam.' I led her up the splendid wooden stairs which the refurbishment had been built around, and I felt a certain pride as I explained the centre was intended to bypass hospitals to make care easy for people, and less expensive. The two bodyguards eyed me without alarm. Had they known what I was capable of thinking they would have frisked me.

Anne's lady-in-waiting had made a prior visit, and so she asked all the right questions. I noticed the awed look in the staff's eyes as they bowed, and how they answered like schoolchildren being examined. In the poly-care clinic a reformed drug addict called Harry asked about her horse, and they shared a turf moment. I restrained myself from telling her that my grandfather ran a mare that *finished* the Grand National and, as I cycled home, not displeased with myself at avoiding an inopportune moment, I composed a verse in my head:

> Her hair was a cobweb
> which at a touch released
> the fly into my eye.
> The spider gouged it out.
> I can't see her baldness.

Joab Comfort didn't like it. 'Embarrassment at being impressed by the Princess Royal makes you petty.'

'It's a comment on inbreeding.'

'By the ill-bred consumed with raw resentments handed down from generation to generation, bemoaning that if only the Spanish Armada had not hit bad weather, and the French hadn't long lunches, the Famine wouldn't have happened, and there would have been an Irish Catholic on the English throne.'

'Up the Republic,' I said, feebly.

'You shouldn't notice bad hair days in women,' I could hear O'Hickee say.

I thought of my raw resentments. My decades in London had healed most of them, and the scars were not visible. One lingered. England made an honest man of me when I could ill-afford it. I arrived on 1 July 1967 and, when registering with the university for further study, I gave the exact date, and had to pay the overseas student rate. Backdated by a month, I would have got free education. Only a fool or me would not have blurred a detail that couldn't be checked.

I suppose I wanted to start my life with the ancient enemy on an honest footing. It meant though that I had to moonlight in makeshift jobs to cover my financial embarrassment. But reflecting back, I wouldn't have wanted to miss out on my days of ordinary madness, particularly for a lie.

RAGS ON THE BUSHES

After my encounter with ambiguity in the Whitechapel cinema, I put together a collage of newspaper cuttings and patriotic quotations that I had collected over the years. I called it 'Conceptual Art and the IRA': 'Two gunmen forced their way into a taxi and fired at the driver and shot each other dead.' I concocted a dialectic of statements made by Orange and Green partisans. '*What we've got to lose is what we've got. The Fenians can only lose a dream.*' (Ulster Unionist, 1980), and '*Those you can't abide, take them to be inanimate objects. You can't alter them, but you can use them sometimes. It's not what they are but what they represent.*' (Republican, 1981). The Hegelian synthesis was an exchange on television between John Hume and Ian Paisley after a debate ended in deadlock. Hume said, '*I'll sleep on it.*' Paisley replied, '*You won't sleep.*'

On a beautiful day in July 1982 I had taken a lunchtime sandwich to the lake in Regent's Park to listen to the army band. Passing the zoo I heard an explosion. I knew the hollow sound from other recent IRA bombings. The Green Jackets had been blown up. I turned back, walking slowly so as not to be considered a suspect, angrily thinking of AE's famous remark. 'Someone should write a play about how for seven hundred years generations fought for the liberation of beautiful Cathleen Ni Houlihan and, when they set her free, out walked a fierce, vituperative old hag.' It was inadequate. I had been looking forward to the music. Deckchairs 25p. I had the coins in my pocket. The collector always made a fuss about change. The concert was routinely attended by pensioners, lunchers from offices in Baker Street, a scatter of tourists, students smooching in the bushes, nannies with prams…

Mindful of my Irish identity, I hesitated. But knew I had to face what Kierkegaard called 'the trial by compassion'. I cycled on into the park. Chaos reigned. The cordon around the inner circle was not yet closed. Police, fearing further bombs, were running sniffer dogs around the lake. The concert programme was pinned to a bower in the rose gardens. Thomas Arne, Verdi, *South Pacific*. When the bomb went off under the bandstand, the

Green Jackets' bandsmen had been tuning up. Not much was left of them, save some rags hanging on the bushes.

On the bridge opposite the bandstand I wrote with a red marker: 'Fire, water, air, stars, sky'. I needed a cloud of Cartesian hope, but it evaporated even before I added 'Virchow lives'.

Cycling home I remembered that a trial by compassion goes against you unless you cast a 'cold eye on life, on death' and ride on. Sometimes it's better to be guilty than innocent.

The following Easter I bumped into Ernie, the deputy head who had befriended me in the days of the school-lunch project. We still met on and off in the Heroes of Alma pub in Maida Vale. His son, who had joined the army because he couldn't pass examinations, was with him. The permanent scars on his fresh face were officially described as facial trauma due to social unrest in Northern Ireland.

Ernie told me the surgeon in the Royal Free Hospital actually used the expression 'Let's face it...' when explaining why the grafts wouldn't take. 'And, I suppose, Andrew has,' he joked helplessly, hopelessly.

The boy had the look of the rags.

PART TWO

V

A PROPER JOB

'All vain tumult and salary.'

—Shakespeare

THE OPEN DOOR

SINCE DEAN SLOWEY'S CAVALRY HAD RESCUED ME FROM peer review (and hadn't mentioned the 'dangerous' clinicians again), my murky career was coasting. I wrote colour pieces for the medical comics, free sheets widely read. I even had my own cartoonist, 'Long', whom I only met on the page. Subjects varied from how to dress and behave on home visits to the wearing of rubber gloves. My style owed something to late Schopenhauer. 'If you want to know if your housebound patient is compos mentis, ask her where she keeps the money. And if she tells you, you know you are in gaga-land.'

I signed them with my mother's family name, always making sure the time I spent on them was commensurate with the minimal wage. This lent a sporting interest. Having recycled a few of the less contentious pieces for pay journals, I realised I was becoming a hack. I strove to make the serious intent more obvious. When I wrote a veiled piece on Virchow, the editor said, 'No politics. It depresses people.' Instead I concocted a piece on the significance of smiles and tears in making a diagnosis, and he said, 'You're getting too personal.' I stopped before I embarrassed myself further by becoming sincere.

Dean Slowey employed me to introduce undergraduates to the history of public health and the ideas behind it. I took them on trips to places of public health pilgrimage, such as Broad Street in Soho where John Snow made the connection between the local water pump and a cholera epidemic. I could communicate better on the hoof. I took them to the British Museum when it was raining. Catching up with the past was a forward march to the Egyptian mummies, where I would talk about the trade in mummy, a medieval cure-all. Dead bodies were embalmed and dried out to make a powder sold to itinerant healers. Virgin mummy was particularly prized, but, like heroin now, it was illegal, and scarce. Traders would kill girls to obtain it. A stash could get your throat cut by a rival healer.

In the canteen, my charges flirted with the foreign refugees from the Reading Room. But students were changing. Some even wore bespoke suits like Consultants. The dressers didn't appreciate my rambles, and spoke of exams and marks. I was complained of for not taking my classes seriously, and Dean the Dean came to see me. As it was a nice sunny day, I had the students sitting outside, and was smoking my pipe. He found himself a chair and joined us.

I had brought along a mechanical calculator, a type of cash register with a bell, which I had picked up in Portobello Market. Leibniz had invented the first modern one three hundred years before. He was my current bathroom reading, and I launched into his idea of creating an alphabet of all human thought, based on symbolic characters. It would establish automatic thinking that would eventually arrive at the indubitable Truth. He abandoned the notion when he realised it would require so many characters that nobody could reasonably expect to keep track of them in order to form words and sentences. The Book of Life would be unreadable.

My bedside reading was Freud, and how he made ends meet. It was prefaced by how famous men from Newton to Marx made a living. Leibniz and Freud had one thing in common. They wanted money, and quick. In their early years they respectively moonlighted in mechanical toys and cocaine (for medical use). When that failed, Freud made his pile on rich patients. Leibniz went for popularising his ideas. But that backfired. He didn't reference his work and bankrupted himself defending his reputation against plagiarism.

If he had gone further with his calculator and invented the first computer, I said, his Book of Life could have been written by high-speed artificial intelligence. He would have paid off his debts, and prospered, as Christ made the Church rich through his disciples dictating the New Testament. Every household once had a Bible and telephone book: the telephone book to get someone else's number, the Bible to get one's own (but of course the truth of the latter is ex-directory).

After initial interest, when I talked about money, the students got restless and I curtailed the class. Dean Slowey suggested that maybe I would be better off just talking to myself. A remark Schopenhauer would have disputed, I replied, but I restrained myself from quoting him. 'Speaking to yourself is imprudent. It establishes thought on such friendly terms with speech that

the gulf between what we say and feel is narrowed. A bad habit.'
Arthur was wrong, the talking in my head said.

I renewed contact with Edna Gray of the Reimbursement
Board, and helped her fine-tune her index on average work-output. Her use of public information was no longer closet. She was
moving it into the mainstream via the Mandarins. The idea of the
bad apples in the barrel of the medical profession was coming to
the fore with insurance companies and legal challenges. Major
scandals were around the corner, she felt certain, looking at
the data with her brilliant eye. Edna didn't really need me, but
the company was welcome. The Reimbursement Board was
beside the sea. I amused her by swimming while smoking my
pipe (lighting it while riding my bike was my ultimate sporting
achievement. Once when pedalling along Canfield Gardens, a
City gent with a bowler and a waxed moustache bowed to me
as I threw away the match).

The door of my murky career had been left open, and something totally unexpected walked in. The Established Order was
being rocked by Mrs Sibyl, a politician who 'raved about as one
possessed hoping to dislodge the mighty god in her bosom'.
At first I felt she was none of my business, a phenomenon of
a decolonised Empire, picking up the pieces. But the return of
Boadicea, armed with a handbag and chain-mailed in a twin-set,
riding into battle on a supermarket trolley, castors spiked with
knives, was a myth in the making. Particularly as she was a blonde
and blue-eyed grocer's daughter with a chemistry degree.

A forgotten colony in the South Atlantic was sent an Armada,
while on the home front coal mines and factories were closing;
the country's underbelly ripped open, and lame ducks dropped
out. The streets became almost Victorian with beggars, tramps

and cripples. England, it was said, was once again a land of opportunity for adventurers willing to take risks.

Deregulation was the watchword, and it came with opportunities. Not least for bankers and entrepreneurs to do what they wanted. Back alleys due for demolition were gentrified. Owning your own house was made easy by mortgage relaxants. Even council houses went on the market. In the borough of Westminster they were seen to attract Sibylline voters. Property was theft, plus politics. At the same time the war against crime concentrated on the dispossessed, who robbed the rich, who robbed everybody else. Security became a growth industry. Doors were double-locked, windows double-glazed.

Mrs Sibyl, lowering her tone, talked about good housekeeping being based on making economies, and wanted to know where the money spent on health went. Previous attempts to get to the bottom of expenditure had failed as accountants came up against its 'historical' basis. Any retrenching was marginalised to what was easiest to cut (eyes and teeth). The Sibyl's attempt gave the accountants the power to dig deeper into the archaeology, but continued to ignore the consequences of economies of convenience. The Mandarins well knew that repairing the likely damage to essential services due to indiscriminative cuts would in the end cost more than the money saved. In the face of ministerial deaf ears, they were concentrating on getting the Established Order to close ranks. The Great and Good were on their dignity, and resisting. The Eminents hesitated. 'Waiting,' Mal Combes said, 'to make up their minds which way to jump.'

The medical domain had been caught off balance. But it regained its equilibrium when it became apparent that Health

was safe for the moment from the general surge towards privatisation. Politically it remained untouchable it seemed. The
exemption came at a price. The health service had been in effect
above money at a grassroots level. Gross national expenditure
was calculated for government budgets, but it wasn't strictly local-
ised, and its itemisation, except in politically sensitive services,
was, to say the least, relaxed. It came as a shock to free-wheeling
managers and free-spending Consultants that the costs had to
be clarified, and in detail. Some trusts were so deep in debt that
they were to form a blacklist of 'failing' services. Panic measures
were in the air.

Politicians talked about value for money. Accountants preferred cost-effectiveness. The civil servants deepened it with
the epidemiological concept of cost-benefit. The negative consequences of withholding care were pointed out. The bottom
line was that it would cost more in the long run. The Sibylites
became thoughtful and, for the time being, prudence was their
watchword. The death of the young wife of a junior minister
during a minor operation in a private clinic, where corners
were being cut with support staff, concentrated their minds.
Cost-benefit analysis offered effective opposition from within.
It provided a baseline for Virchow, I thought. Health before
politics. I wanted to be part of it. 'Failed' services were to be my
point of entry.

By then, I was more or less accepted as someone who would
not go away. The peer review initiative had normalised the
clinical audit of services. My part in the early stages had been
noted and, according to Mal Combes, I was on a list of potential
troubleshooters along with a motley crew of petty tyrants, some
from industries which had failed.

Meanwhile, Dean Slowey's fears for patients would have to be addressed, I knew. I had already handed over the names of the 'dangerous' clinicians picked up in peer review for Edna to compare her pay data to, and she confirmed there was enough complementary evidence in several cases for disciplinary proceedings to be recommended, if supported by complaints. Whether Edna's information could be used at the hearing was doubtful. The Medical and Dental associations would be up in arms, threatening god-knows-what.

Cassandra of Human Resources warned me that with high-paid professionals, and their expensive lawyers, rather than union representatives, I would be entering the inner circle of hell. This couldn't be avoided in clear-cut cases of criminal negligence. Indeed one of our 'dangerous' clinicians appeared to have been successfully dealt with by the trust that employed him. The alternative I suggested to Dean Slowey was radical. If the law of the land could be invoked for cases of 'criminal negligence', surely it could be extended to 'gross incompetence' (currently left to the tender mercy of the Medical Council). All it needed was for the government to make minor changes in the law. I said that with rising insurance claims it would be inevitable. 'Welcome to America,' he sighed. But he remained sceptical. 'The councils would never relinquish control.'

Using Edna's index on peer review groups with known 'errants' (a less tabloid-damning term than 'quacks' or 'horse doctors') I proposed instead a Mandarin-backed study. His researchers would jump at it. Ethical approval for the study could be obtained without recourse to the Medical Council. I waxed lyrical and said, if Virchow were to come into being, it would have to be accountable to the common weal, and not to professional bodies and their politicians. 'Keep that under your hat or, better still, eat it,' was his reply.

But it was all happening. Research spin-offs from Dean Slowey's peer review were taken up as topics for doctoral students. Mal Combes and Dean the Dean were working in tandem. I made available the raw data from my master file. As some of this research had a public-interest dimension, on Mal Combes's prompting, the Great and Good invited me to local Health Authority meetings. It gave me something to do. If my presentation was favourably received, I shyly mentioned Virchow. Although it drew cynical laughs, the idea of a health-driven worldview had indubitable appeal. One chairperson solemnly declared, 'It's the ideal we are all moving towards.'

THE TROUBLESHOOTER

Mal Combes cautioned me, 'Once you're considered a good thing, then people start finding you indispensable, meaning the opposite, and offer you jobs nobody wants. You find you can't refuse them. Flattery's secret weapon, Poet, is it pricks one's vanity, and you end up with your own blood on your hands.' And sure enough, the Mandarins invited me to the department, and I found myself part of the motley troupe of troubleshooters for 'failing' trusts.

The mystery Mandarin of the Soho lunch did the talking. 'These trusts are not "failing" because of poor clinical performance, but more the tradition of spending their money as though there's no tomorrow. Now a fixed budget has to be adhered to. However we mustn't throw out the baby with the bath water.

Cuts when they're indiscriminate won't save lives or money. Cost-benefit considerations are the only prudent way forward. Persuading the Powers That Be that this is so is the other side of the troubleshooter's job.' Thanks to Mrs Sibyl, I was no longer on the outside looking in and, to my surprise, in the inner sanctum the longview taken by Descartes, Virchow and common sense, had a voice. This was music to my ears, but was it just a serenade?

I was entering a disaster area. The world outside was impatient. Politicians wanted it now, the now that would keep them in power. As did the Ground Forces, the now that they knew. Reconciling them wasn't really possible. I had some experience of trying to redeem lost causes from my Ordinary Madness days with Dr McCall and Jo Manders. Then I was dealing with ingenious paradoxes. Now it was a cauldron of contradictions. However, mindful of Coleridge's 'Work without hope draws nectar in a sieve/and hope without an object cannot live', I banked on enlightened self-interest. Money was what they had in common. If they could see its beneficial use was its only true value, maybe the impasse could be broken. That was closer to Leibniz's *optimisme* than Descartes's down-to-earth hope, but at least I had an objective.

'Disasters teach you all you need to know about people,' Roger Toussaint of Accident and Emergency liked to say. I wasn't so sure. The Mandarins bypassing the Eminents augured ill for them in a small way. I was invited to the group to discuss things. Nothing really was said that wasn't already known. The unsaid was that I had not consulted them. But their change in attitude to me wasn't subtle. I was no longer an *enthusiast* for Stanley O. Kay. I was a loose cannon. The sneer king of the group, Max Madison, still mocked me as Mal Combes's Fool:

'He that has but a little tiny wit,
  With heigh-ho, the wind and the rain,
  Must make content with his fortune fit.'

I knew my place.

Lingering at the door, I could hear Dame Brenda drone on in full pomp and titters of laughter. But I couldn't make out a word. No doubt she was flying a kite about me, mixing metaphors with vulgarities to keep her Yorkshire feet on the ground. Something like, 'Mal Combes's whipping boy's promotion to being the clown in a failing circus where the ring-master is quietly going bats, should be worth the entrance fee. When the Big Top is blown down he will be left standing in the sawdust waving his political naïvety. Our pet Paddy is setting himself up to fail. Mal can't protect him any more. At the first false step he makes, it's gotcha.'

Maybe she was just talking about Shakespeare, not me. How the Fool's ditty in *King Lear* is not a song about himself, as the King assumed, but a wistful comment on his majesty's state of mind. I wouldn't be making a compliment out of the gibe, but it was true that my elective 'king' was being driven mad by the new generation of Consultants, amongst them the younger Eminents. They had begun to veto Mal Combes's interventions in Upper Echelon matters. The wily old fox, Stanley O. Kay, was said to be behind it. I pumped Mal Combes. He shrugged his shoulders. 'The brat Eminents are more likely to oust him. His cultured air is a cover for grounding himself in the past, and doing as little as possible. I've a better head for the dizzy heights than poor Stanley.'

I knew that many of the young Consultants had been students of his, and once he got working on them they would come around. I had to believe that. I depended on Mal Combes. He was my safety net. If I was pushed from a height, I would soft-land and bounce back. Or should I go too far and hit a glass ceiling, he would pick me up, give me a dusting down and, if I agreed to go quietly, make sure I was paid off in kind: the Mandarins would be told who pushed me.

I felt for the first time in my working life that I was swimming in the mainstream, and I was damned if the likes of Dame Brenda and Max Madison, would jeer from the banks as they watched me drown. I would stay on dry land, and watch those I was supposed to be struggling with in the cross currents. The ground was moving under me, but that kept me on my toes. If I was going to be caught it would have to be on the hop.

Resolutions are the brave face that confronts the weak one in the mirror. I cycled to where my fellow troubleshooters for the region were being briefed. I had discovered the Grand Union Canal and its towpaths, so I didn't have to negotiate the London traffic. Pedalling pensively calmed my nerves, and by the time I arrived at the department I achieved what Epicurus called ataraxia: a mind emptied in order to attain stoical indifference. All the better to take in what was expected of me.

The 'failing' trust's finances were presented. The bottom line was clear, but the rest was a mammoth mess. It was necessary to talk to the finance manager to find out where the money was going. He identified the heavy-spending hospitals and health centres. And so I took to my bike again to visit them. Everywhere I went the staff were too busy to talk to me. I didn't see any conspicuous waste. On the Grand Union Canal I sat on a bench listening to Schubert songs on my Walkman ('Only the desolate can know my sorrow'), and contemplating my reflection in the murky waters. I would have to go deeper into the data.

The trust offered me my own office and two fifths of a secretary. But I chose to return to my converted toilet where I could hide out. I rejected the dainty morsel of a secretary, using the typing pool wherever I found myself. I got to know the girls by first names. I'm not sure they ever quite knew who, or what, I was, because my name wasn't on the trust telephone lists.

When someone asked 'Who is he?' they said, 'one of Professor Combes's assistants,' for I copied most of my letters to him. I don't think they took in the content of my correspondence, which was largely functional, confirming some verbal agreements, or memos received. What I put on paper I kept to the minimal. Though sometimes I wrote up the minutes of tempestuous meetings to limit the waffle, and then had to be careful who typed it out. I tended to use secretaries who responded to my O'Hickee hair compliment with a smile. They knew what was important.

Even the Eminents began to wonder whose Trojan Horse I was. I had been seen lunching with Dean Slowey, and appeared to spend more time in the Department of Health than them (that was because a junior Mandarin had just completed his doctoral thesis on cost-benefit, and I was reading it with him in order to pick his brains). However, the Eminents had reason to regard me as a 'loose cannon'. They knew I had chosen to be on a contract that didn't include bonuses, which meant I had no line manager. I could come and go as I pleased. It was like being my own boss, and I worked my own hours.

The Eminents asked to see my job description, and I said I hadn't written it yet. Dame Brenda raised the matter of a conflict of interest. 'You're still working within the trusts on behalf of Dean Slowey, and at the same time being paid by the department.' So she knew about my follow-up probes with peer review groups but, fortunately, not Edna Gray. I said, 'No. I've resigned as the projects person.' She wanted to know who I was accountable to. I wanted to say to the devil and the Minister of Health, the same as you. Instead, I said, 'It's still in the process of clarification.' Max Madison heaved in: 'It is a case of power without responsibility.' That confused me. I had responsibilities and no visible power. So, to throw the cat amongst the pigeons, I said, 'If I had my way I would be accountable to the Eminents Group.' That did not displease them. But, as the group dispersed, I knew I had further distanced myself from being one of them, because Max Madison patted me on the back.

THE CUTTING EDGE

After the period of obstinate stropping with the peer review groups, and the minor dash I cut when it was taken up by Dean Slowey, ambiguity was returning and I was living on a moral edge. Milton's 'double sense of deluding' honed it to razor sharpness. As a troubleshooter I could be seen as a hit man or a saint of cost-benefit. But I was neither nor. I was a debt collector for a government with an ideology that said health is money.

The talking in my head was impatient with me. 'Turn the blade against yourself then,' it said. 'The closer to drawing blood the better. You will be living a metaphor, rendering your body hairless to smooth your way like a racing cyclist in cross-winds. Nobody need see you speed past. You're a specialist in lone breaks, not a part of the peloton. Spin off or stay put, depending on the circumstances. Be your mother's son.'

In effect, I was just a functionary with a paperknife. I settled down to the task in hand. It was all perspiration and no inspiration. I was sweating over facts and figures to slim them down to bottom lines. I was getting the details right, a servant to the devil. When I broke for a breather I avoided people's eyes. I wore the same clothes, but what was inside them was below talking temperature. I would let the facts speak for themselves.

Deciphering information was like dissection. I was getting under the trust's skin to make my imprint from the inside. It was cold-blooded work. I had to be incisive. Otherwise I'd only be scratching the surface. I cut clean, and deep. The surgery was not cosmetic: designed to save face or blushes, either mine, or in the body of the evidence. I worked close to the bone, evading arteries to avoid spillage, extracting foreign bodies with a forceps, exposing each dossier to the light, and checking it for false tracks, bringing dead facts to life.

Making it a metaphor makes it more interesting, I suppose. It was for the most part deadly boring. Still my task was to see if the figures added up, and find the cause of the deficit. I looked beyond money to clinical work-output, and the performance there was distinctly healthy. That suggested, since some of the best peer review groups were in this 'failing' trust, that clinical standards were higher than average. In short, the Ground Forces were caught in the friendly fire between mismanagement and the Powers That Be. They would suffer collateral damage as the walls of fixed budgets closed in on them.

The managers regarded me as a sinister intrusion, and not surprisingly they played possum, or froze me out. The most invisible of them was the chief executive. Harry Huggins was old school, used to respect and dinners in County Hall. He locked his office door against what he called the new dispensation, and passed messages to the outside world through his ancient secretary, whose competence did not include the sharing of confidences. Once I finished my dissection of the body of evidence, I wanted to see him. But I didn't get past his secretary. In a note he suggested I occupy myself with identifying practical concerns like the crumbling infrastructure. I could see why the politicians were in favour of blanket cuts.

Mindful of the Madison pat, I confided my findings to the Eminent Persons Group, concluding that controlling the expenditure of money so it could be more beneficially redistributed would be difficult with the current chief executive. My confidence put them on first-name terms with me, but I could not bring myself to call them Brenda, Max and Stanley. I left as promptly as I could, feeling they had got what they wanted, a submission. And Mal Combes would not be best pleased at my two-timing.

But the very next day he came to see me. This was unheard of. At best I could expect a phone call. The visit wasn't to pillory me. Now that Una was safely married, and Nasty had started on Proust, despite his problems with the Upper Echelons, he was in rousing form. 'You look as though you're in a Greek tragedy. But it's only a farce.' I began to pour out my woes, and he stopped me. 'You thought you'd trip them up with Harry Huggins, but it was you that was the fall guy. They will go straight to Harry, and sort something out with him. Then report your indiscretion to the Mandarins, and the show will go on. Nobody will pay any attention to you.'

'So I'm wasting my time.'

'That's what time is for, my friend. But you can make it interesting. Stand at the back and marvel at what is being enacted. It's a play within a play. The deeper you dig the more the plot thickens. Take your list of managers. Only Harry Huggins's name is known to me. But Roger Black could turn out to be an ex-Nazi. Trevor White an international conman. Susie Calder *was* a man. Harry, by the way, is as Irish as you. Yet he behaves like John Bull himself, though I believe nowadays he's more like a lamb to the slaughter. Ask MacCrone's advice.'

Mal Combes was off before I could ask 'Who is MacCrone?'

I wouldn't be investigating the background of the managers. The talking in my head said my troubleshooting mustn't become personal. Neither would I be playing to the gallery with the Mandarins. Election year was looming, and the less they saw of me, the more they liked me. I might have a quick word with them in passing in the corridors of power. My verbal floats were well understood, and the response signalled was hierarchical. If a top civil servant smiles and shakes your hand briskly it means 'Yes, I approve'. If he looks you in the eye blankly, it's a 'No. Go away'. If the head is inclined to the left it means 'I'm thinking about it'. An incline to right is 'Is that what you think?' and, if followed by a short laugh, 'you're on board'. Not a word has been spoken, but speech melodies are not necessary. Should he sign off by turning to someone else, you know he's too busy for the likes of you. Frankness may be all, but it cannot be quoted.

MacCrone rang (he was the mystery Mandarin), and told me to make my reports to the Health Authority from now on. 'They are the money.' Health Authorities decided what funds would be made available to trusts to provide services in their area. Their members were government appointees, but they had expert executive support. Public Health was central, and its director, Angela Khan, had been co-opted from Dean Slowey's teaching hospital. After a short lunch in Paddington Station I found that I had become one of her advisors. It wasn't just Dean's recommendation. My days of Ordinary Madness had given me an *entrée* by the backdoor. When trusts requested approval for atypical treatments related to the head and neck, and hepatitis B, I was faxed.

My troubleshooter reports to the Health Authority were without metaphors: point-blank facts and figures. I left the Eminents to present them at meetings. I wouldn't want the Great and Good to think I was a lapsed idealist. I got the odd enquiry from local papers and radio. But I certainly was not going to play to the gods. The general public was somewhere out there in the dark, and there they would stay, mostly sitting quietly, and clapping when the curtains went down. 'Not much is happening,' I told the journalists. 'Keep in touch.'

'Not hitting the headlines, Poet,' said Mal Combes, 'will disappoint Dame Brenda, and please the Mandarins. "Health trust boss locks himself in his office and takes secretary as a hostage" would put you on the spot. What's happening, or not, is best kept as an open secret.'

Mal Combes's working life was a play within a play within a play. I asked myself did he want to prick consciences and, if so, who was the king? Could it be himself? But as a royal person he was closer to Lear than Hamlet, being often decisively wrong. I was not unhappy to be called his Fool by Max. However, Una as his Cordelia would be miscast. But not Nasty as his mother. It could only end badly, except for Mal Combes. He would be doubling up as Fortinbras.

WHAT EXACTLY WAS GOING ON?

One lives forwards and thinks backwards, Kierkegaard says. I try to recapture what was going through my head. How could I? At the time clarity was an emotion that came and went with circumstances not always under my control. Afterthoughts tend towards embellishment. A conjectural reconstruction is all that can be promised. Like a free-jazz musician with an old standard, I improvise, testing the notes for the ring of truth, and always find them wanting.

The hard facts are easier on the memory. What I was doing was officially ambiguous. I was there to help 'failing' services to fail better and advise the moneybags on cost-benefit. This gave me a dual presence. I was working on both sides of the moon. But the only real power I had was in my verbal floats to those who made the decisions. If my advice was taken I had only myself to blame. Whereas with peer review, when the decisions were made by clinicians on the ground, I felt virtuous.

Political intrusion became more brutal approaching elections. Bureaucratic panic set in when politicians in power began to harass their civil servants. Realising that quality cannot be guaranteed – there would always be still-born babies discovered in laundries – promoting quantity was the command. A rise in tonsillectomies or hip replacements could swing the vote. Mrs Sibyl was much taken by the Oregon (USA) referendum to bring popular choice into public spending on Health. In effect, money was diverted to surgical procedures that affect the largest number of people, such as wisdom-teeth removal and hip replacements. The joke was that when you heard an ambulance siren, 'there goes another ingrown toenail.'

MacCrone, after delivering a press statement, bemoaned, 'One has to appear to be carrying the donkey while at the same time riding it.' Aesop's *Fables* was his consolation, and the fact that after the hue and cry it would be back to doing what he wanted. I wasn't so sure. Mrs Sibyl had titled her first white paper on health 'Patients First'. Thus waging war on all those who saw the health of the population as the priority. Several bright young epidemiologists threw in the towel and joined the pharmaceutical industry, where they probably did more harm than good, and now sail round the world in their yachts.

Furthermore, she announced, without consulting the Mandarins, that trusts don't have to 'fail'. The private sector and teaching hospitals would come to their rescue. Her junior health minister hinted independent trusts were the model for the future, meaning privatisation. The reverse of Virchow was in train: sickness as the norm, and for profit. My guiding light had no place in this world. Medicine was politics on a slippery slope. Declaring the National Health Service 'safe in my hands', she was re-elected with a comfortable majority.

Except perhaps to Mrs Sibyl, it wasn't a surprise. Her chancellor had been loosening up the economy in a 'dash for growth'. Monetarism had been quietly dropped, and unemployment fell. But inflation was on the rise, and that made the good housekeeper in her anxious. Still, her victory was assured by the opposition leader, an intellectual, who was said to be 'out of touch' with reality. I used to see him on Hampstead Heath walking the dog, with his Byronic limp and white, windswept mane. His manifesto included banning fox hunting and nuclear weapons. Worst of all, he appeared to be wearing a donkey jacket at the Cenotaph on Remembrance Day.

HARRY HUGGINS'S HEAVY MANTLE

When Harry Huggins finally opened the door of his office, it was to commit himself to a mental hospital. I agreed to act up until someone was appointed. Cassandra told me that wouldn't be for some time. The finance manager wanted the post frozen to save money. So I was to be offered a two-year contract. Not as a deputy chief executive. That would need an interview. After much bureaucratic soul-searching the title arrived at was acting head of services, with intimations of mine being put on the block. The salary was set at the equivalent to a senior manager.

Pressure was mounting. MacCrone rang to say that a feasibility study on the new independent model was underway. Business consultants were leading it. Fears of a 'Harley Street takeover' would be more real without someone who knew the trust, and who the trust knew, in place. Newfangled managers from industry, or retired from the armed forces, were coming into vogue. I would be the lesser evil. I resigned as a troubleshooter, and accepted the job with a heavy heart. 'Accidents of destiny' were determining my life, 'and they are not conducive to creative work' (Yves Bonnefoy). I could forget Vichow.

Passing Mal Combes's garden, he came to the gate. 'Got yourself a proper job. My commiserations.' He tapped the back of his gardening glove against my hand. 'Getting things done in a cash-strapped trust, Poet, and doing for yourself, could be one and the same thing.'

I was required by employment law to have management training, and took a weekend course in South Kensington. The Franciscan-like guru (beard and sandals) gently concluded the final seance, 'All good management, like life and death, is exit

148

management. You suffer for some time before you go to your reward.' This analogy appealed to me and, taking my cue from this wise man, I swore I would never wear the suit and tie. The bike would be my alibi. I girded my loins for what was ahead.

Needless to say, the Eminents raised the matter of a conflict of interest, and it couldn't be denied there was one. I could have stood my ground, saying that I only gave advice; the Health Authorities could take it or leave it. But I knew conflict of interest would haunt my new job. I spoke to MacCrone. 'You'll have to go undercover. The surest way to arrange that is not to officially resign, but to get fired. After that, there's nothing stopping them ringing you up for advice.'

One lingering failure in peer review was in cross-infection control. Resistance to change was widespread despite increased funding to cover the cost. This was most noticeably evident amongst old-school surgeons (often be-knighted) who had private practices in Harley and Wimpole Street. When passing by, you could still see boiling-water sterilisers through the windows. No doubt for instruments used in minor surgery. In the wake of hepatitis B and HIV, and with a clientele that included high-risk groups such as pop stars, this was criminal, I thought. Even tattooists had moved on.

When a senior dental nurse from the trust who worked Saturdays in a private practice reported that injection needles were being re-used, without consulting anybody, not even Mal Combes, I phoned the morning radio talk-show host, and offered to take calls on clinical hygiene. At breakfast time I spoke to Londoners on what they should expect of doctors and dentists in order to protect them from viruses that could kill. 'It is a mistake to think like George Bernard Shaw that the medical profession is in conspiracy against the public. All you have to do is ask. The next time you have an appointment pose the following questions on their equipment and procedures...'

A flood of complaints to the Medical and Dental councils ensued. I received a warning from both councils that I was bringing their professions into disrepute. The Health Authority disowned me, or rather let it be known I was no longer an advisor. I got a call from Angela Khan of Public Health ticking me off, but adding, 'Off the record, you did what we all would have loved to do. I will keep in touch.'

My questions were pirated on a poster by the Health Education Department and officially circulated for display in waiting rooms. I suppose I was an anarchist of hygiene. But the impulse I indulged in not only freed me from accusations of a conflict of interest, it was in a way an indication that in my new job I was capable of anything to make things that ought to happen happen, and also some things that ought not.

Mal Combes came to see me again with more theatrical advice: 'You were never intended, Poet, to take centre stage. But now that you're Harry Huggins's stand-in, I've come to rehearse you: keep your storyline to yourself. Let the plot dawn on your audience gradually. Concentrate on the stage details. That's where the devil is. It's what's noticed. Get it wrong, and people stamp their feet and whistle... First, get to know the supporting cast – all the staff, no matter how humble. For a genuine ensemble you have to go beyond the brainstorming egoists who think they run the show. The spear carriers and the walk-ons are not usually allowed to speak. But they are the whispering chorus to the motleys who do the shouting. And don't forget to credit them with names. It's no mean task getting them right, but well worth the effort. James not Jim. Miss Brown not Sally. The secretaries will know. However, remain "Doctor" yourself, except at out-of-hours meetings. After that, it is usually enough to keep a hooded eye on goings-on, and play by Human Resources. They'll tell you what you can get away with. Exit, pursued by a bear.'

Cassandra laughed at Mal Combes's advice. 'London is a Babel. You'll find your staff speak forty different languages, fortunately not all at the same time. The cleaners are mostly Spaniards; the porters, West Indians; the orderlies, illegal immigrants; the auxiliaries, refugees from Africa and South America. There will be a smattering of odd bods including a token transvestite (ours is Jerry). Clerks and receptionists are a United Nations of divorcees, widows and one-parent families; nurses, Irish and Caribbean; the professionals, a four-leaf clover of Celts, Jews, Asians, and some English; middle management, mainly ex-nurses and university graduates who couldn't find jobs in their chosen subject. I'm one of them. There is some upward mobility, but not at the top. The Consultants are almost exclusively male and white as the royal family.'

THE BIG PUSH

I was already working up what to say to staff. 'You have the pick of clinicians in the country, and yet you are seen as failures. This is based on performance targets set up from national averages. The problem is you are not average. London is a Mecca for all the health problems in the world. People flood in here with conditions that haven't a conventional fix. Day by day, you have to deal with refugees, asylum seekers, homeless people, drug addicts, and other lost souls, and in over forty different languages.

'And yet it is rumoured that you are to become guinea pigs for seismic changes that nobody is going to like. You are piggy-in-the-middle between the devil of funding and the deep blue sea of privatisation. What's to be done? It's time for a Big Push to show to the world what you demonstrate so effectively with your patients. Nobody wants you to 'fail' except the government.'

I was embarrassed by my own rhetoric. Actions speak. Talk does not act. I needed to express myself without the noise of words. I heard music wafting from the estates manager's office. Duke Ellington's 'Do Nothing till You Hear from Me'. I found a pretext to visit Jim Barrett. Not to interrupt the 'piano cocktail', but to sit quietly for a minute.

'Duke is my lifeline,' he whispered. 'The art of the ellipsis.'

'A musical litotes,' I whispered back, 'He leaves out notes, but you hear them.'

When the tape ended, Jim said, 'When Miles Davis asked Duke how he managed to make his big band of drunks, junkies and wife beaters play so harmoniously, he replied 'I never let them disturb my beautiful temperament' (a phrase I've used ever since as a litotes of mine).

My pretext was to get a map of the trust's properties. And Jim Barrett gave me an idea. The trust had properties of untold value underused or vacant in central London. They could be put on the market and the money used to avoid cuts. For instance, there was a disused hospital. This could be refurbished to attract Bright Young Specialists in order to perform elective surgery, largely exclusive to hospitals, in the community, and at one-tenth the cost. In other words I would be taking on the teaching hospitals.

Unheard of, except it happened to be Dean Slowey's suggestion when I phoned him.

'Only a fool or you,' said Mal Combes, borrowing my catch-phrase. 'Do you realise that all the Medical Council will be on your tail? And Harley Street won't like the competition from the public sector. But enemy number one will be the hospital Consultants. You will be poaching on their territory. Not since Nye Bevan have they faced such a challenge.'

Mal Combes exaggerated, but he was not displeased. He knew his Bright Young Specialists were the future. They had no time for the trial by sherry that preceded being anointed a Consultant. It was enough to be one in all but name. Their Established Order was in Europe, where the hierarchy was more merit-based. They taught summer courses in Spain and Italy.

'But, bizarrely, Poet, you'll not only have the Mandarins on your side, but the Sibylites too. They'll be all for a business initiative which saves the government money. True, it doesn't accord with their independent trust notion. But there are other "failing" trusts around that can be dismantled for that.' Mal Combes wasn't going to allow me to get carried away. 'Be warned,' he said. 'If your idea is seen as a success, others will take it up and ruin it.' Though he was careful to add, 'Report progress back to me before talking to the Eminents. I'll keep the Mandarins informed. I leave the Health Authority to you. You have Angela Khan in your pocket, as Dame Brenda says.' I thought of the store Santa in *Miracle on 34th Street* who believed in himself until others began to. I felt a fraud.

When I visited Angela Khan we talked of something else. Already my informal advisory role risked exposure. Harley Street had an undue number of clinicians whose failed treatments ended up in the public sector. Often the cases were cosmetic surgery, and cost the earth, twice over. Complaints against a recidivist of botched nose jobs had reached a point when the Health Authority was asking the Medical and Dental Councils to discipline him. The problem was I would be called as a witness. I spoke to Dean Slowey, and he proposed instead that the private errants be brought into clinical audit with my Bright Young Specialists once they got going. There the matter rested.

ONLY ACTING

Mal Combes (and myself) were not the only compulsive users of metaphors. Dame Brenda, when she learnt my conflict of interest had been resolved, said, 'so at last we're singing from the same hymn sheet.' I had a vision of a choir of fallen angels and redeemed devils belting out different words out of tune. And in the wings an ex-holy terror stamping his feet, out of step with the beat. Unison was not my thing.

'Well done,' said Stanley O. Kay. 'And hats off for your promotion. I hope you're not a victim of your own success.'

'Not quite a promotion,' Max Madison intervened. 'His elevation flatters to deceive. He's only "acting" till the real thing comes along.'

'You are setting yourself up to fail all on your own,' Dame Brenda sighed. 'I thought it would be with Mal Combes.'

'I believe he's in the Middle East recruiting sheiks' children as high-paying overseas students in London,' sniggered Max Madison.

'Moving with the times,' chortled Stanley O. Kay.

'"Acting" is an apt title for you,' Dame Brenda darted.

Max Madison tapped me on the shoulder, 'Arise Sir Acting Manager.'

The younger Eminent Persons remained silent. I think they wondered was I on the way up? It wasn't so much the poisoned chalice I found myself holding, but my friendship with Dean Slowey mystified them. Moreover, the autonomy of the group isolated them from what seemed to be happening, and they felt in danger of being left behind by the Bright Young Specialists. Even the name of the group was against them in Mrs Sibyl's specious surge towards egalitarianism. If disbanded, all they could look forward to was their happy band being sucked back into the Consultants' mixing of the poisoned bowl, while the grey Eminents would be kicked upstairs to the House of Lords.

A PHILOSOPHIC INTERLUDE

But I was no longer my own man. I was The Man for numerous needy health workers (I never actually counted them as a slave-driver would). The Brunetial solipsist in me revolted, and reversed Jeremy Bentham's lone prison watch: the trust was my Panopticon tower, but the surveillance had been reversed, and the cells were keeping me under constant observation.

I was a quagmire of muddy emotions. Was I wading in this cesspool to experience why Virchow was necessary, or to satisfy my vanity? Neither struck me as true. I was the victim of an accident rather than success. The only idea in my head when Harry Huggins crashed out was that a vacuum needed to be filled before it imploded, and my honest brokering amongst the trust's facts and figures made me well-informed enough to fill the gap. But I wasn't cut out to be a manager of people, as Mal Combes well knew. A manipulator perhaps, but that was hit and run, and I could make a clean getaway, leaving behind at worst some broken flowers. Now what was expected of me was to stand trial for the accident that I was the victim of. The talking in my head was saying nothing.

Before the mad aria there is always a recitative. I had a few weeks until taking up the appointment. In those null, mercifully dull, days the maze I was in became a familiar place. It was more like a game of bagatelle, and I was the ball slotting into the holes. I went to *Faust* at the Electric Cinema Club, but the silent movie didn't speak to me. The only bargain I had made was with myself.

I needed a period of perfect blankness like when I took to studying after an ill-spent childhood. Ataraxia clears the head. But it's difficult to keep the mind quiet when you have nothing to do. The mind needed to be stretched to the point where I could not think. Philosophy always did that with me. I searched out my Nietzsche and Schopenhauer. They cheered me up.

Schopenhauer was like opening the Bible at random to tell you what to do. 'Life may be hell but you always find a corner to make music.' I played my violin for the first time since the days of Ordinary Madness. My fingers fumbled the notes but I could hear a melodious echo from the past. And it would have pleased my father. I scratched out some double-stopping.

Arthur brought me back to work. 'Everything is fleeting, only change endures', was salutary. I would be a fleeting catalyst of enduring change, but by definition I would be unchanged myself. I would endure. His assurance that 'experience leads to clarity – clearing away the phantoms of the brain that youth conjures', made me wonder was Virchow just a youthful illusion? But still I had only discovered him when I was middle-aged.

His dictum, 'politeness is to human nature what warmth is to wax', made me want to jump up and make my manners to everyone I met on the street. I could perform my acting role with a polite smile on my face. Then I thought of Nietzsche. When he presented himself for treatment for neurosis, the doctor said, 'There is nothing wrong with your nerves, it's me that's nervous.' The doctor was my staff. I felt much better.

ALL THINGS TO ALL

I didn't change my working habits. I cycled to work, keeping the converted toilet as my office, but not to receive people. I went to see them. This was partly influenced by Nye Bevan who, according to his private secretary, didn't summon staff to his office but walked down the corridor, and knocked on your door. But also it allowed me the freedom to get up and leave without being overtly rude. I used the typing pool, but now officially. I chose Michelle of Chinese extraction from French Central Africa to make appointments, take phone calls and oversee my typing. She had come to England when her husband had sued the government over a factory leak that contaminated his family, killing his father and sister. After that he found it difficult to get work. Whether it was a case of politics or not, I don't know, but when I explained Virchow to her she wept.

The typing was in the hands of Ninette, an eager-to-please West Indian girl, who had been on the point of being disciplined for making so many mistakes. On retraining, she showed a remarkable aptitude for audio typing. She heard words better than she read them. Michelle, whose spelling and grammar were impeccable, corrected her letters. The collaboration was mutually agreeable, and I could count on their discretion.

Unobtrusively, I assumed my role. I didn't dress, or behave, the part. This was not as rare in London as elsewhere. I had observed from the younger Consultants it was chic to be casual. Informality relaxed people without compromising respect. A calm descended wherever I went, I liked to think.

I forewent a bumper meeting of staff to introduce myself. Apart from delivering the wrong message by eating into clinical time, rising murmurs of dissent could be expected as the more articulate turned my Big Push into a polemic without issue. My beautiful temperament wouldn't have warmed to that by waxing polite. I could hear myself saying that, after all, making things happen as they ought to was the least that could be expected. Less than that was just slacking. The meltdown would have been nuclear.

Instead, using my troubleshooting data, I visited key clinicians in their workplace at lunch break, bringing my own sandwich, and saying the same thing to each. In sum, do you like your job? And, if so, do you want to keep it? Both questions could hardly be answered in the negative, and so I could go on to outline what was necessary to make themselves indispensable, and avoid cuts. 'See me as your advocate, not your boss.' It worked more often than not, leaving us feeling better about one another.

The democratic approach made more of an impression than if a *deus ex machina* descended and interviewed everybody in an extravagantly redecorated office. I was just like them, in the

same boat. But, as my down-to-earthness replaced fear and deference with confidences and cosy complicity, I downplayed the
crisis the trust was in. My Big Push moderated itself to friendly
nudges, persistent but not too dramatic. In terms of Kierkegaard's
trial by compassion, opting for the soft-soap approach rather
than the hard-nosed has its risks. Confronted by danger on the
road, hesitation leads to stepping back in order to run on the
spot, a left-footed way of staying in the same place. But the
Powers That Be would not accept staying in the same place.
Still, I couldn't bring myself to take the easy way out with a
crass, 'let's face it.'

I planned a monthly newsletter as a way of avoiding meetings.
Ad hoc encounters in corridors, or on the street, could be more
useful. For the time being I limited group gatherings to peer
review sessions linked to refresher courses in resuscitation, or
to demonstrations of some technical advance. I hadn't forgotten
about putting proven solutions into practice.

I had already identified from my rounds the leading live-
wires and/or trouble-makers, and invited them to after-hours
aperitifs. I encouraged free expression, and laughter to go with
it. As long as I didn't try to control them, these occasions were
a congenial forum to offload frustrations, and generate ideas. I
mentioned casually that, all going well, I might consider away-
days in summer before the school holidays. A trip to London
Zoo or even Calais to buy wine. Someone suggested such trips
could be funded by selling waste products. Dental nurses led the
way by collecting silver amalgam. The secretaries followed with
waste paper. Recycling could be profitable.

For the moment, I was answerable to nobody except myself.
The Mandarins had better things to do, cleaning up after Mrs

Sibyl's nervousness before her lucky victory in the general election. No news is good news, as my mother said. Mrs Sibyl no
longer raved like one possessed. 'First the severity of the ideal,
then gentleness,' says Kierkegaard. Her gentleness was heavy-
handed: 'Pippa's Song' crossed with Dr Pangloss. *All was right in
the best of all possible worlds*. The tabloids acted as her Candide.

Human Resources was knocking at my door, overwhelming
me with a backlog of disciplinary cases. Some cases were clear: a
cook who served bad meat in the geriatric ward, a secretary who
made daily transatlantic calls to her personal mystic, a needle
thief caught in the act, a nurse who punched her doctor. But
for the most part the evidence hadn't been properly collected.
Further investigation would open a can of worms. Persuading
errants to resign would be preferable. However that was dangerously close to constructive dismissal. There was no end to the
rope I had inherited.

The most pressing was the maxillofacial surgeon, Lovecraft,
who could only operate before midday as he was alcoholic.
Stanley O. Kay rang me to say, 'Leave it to the Consultants to
sort out. They like to deal with their own. Otherwise…' I knew
he meant I'd be called before the Medical Council, but for what
I wasn't sure. But the Lovecraft case was coming to a head with
mounting complaints from theatre staff over erratic behaviour,
and from families over cancelled operations. However, Edna
Gray came to my rescue. Her index showed he had lower than
average repeat operations, and nothing in his performance profile suggested malpractice. So I had no compunction in ceding
to Stanley.

I accidentally-by-mistake met Lovecraft coming out of theatre, and said, 'I'm going for a pint, why not join me?' He was

only too eager. But he knew I wanted to talk to him. It was easy because I liked him, an agreeable Welshman, who wasn't in denial about his weakness. He ordered a large whiskey and drank it down more or less in one gulp, saying, 'That's better.' We both laughed, but he wasn't joking. I explained my dilemma. I had a management problem with him but not a clinical one. So there was no question of a disciplinary case. He commiserated with me, promptly resigned, and was back in practice within a few months in Harley Street.

By great good fortune I knew the trade union man from my Anarchist Society days. Or rather Dick Cross claimed to remember me. Widely respected for his good-humoured judgements, his role was polyvalent, covering the Ground Forces and the Underlings but also helping out the Medical and Dental associations on an informal basis. Some cases could be sorted amicably with his help. For instance, cases that had been so long pending that the original problem had been rectified or the employee eased into more suitable work. The laundry, ambulance, and kitchen services were invaluable for such transfers with lower-paid staff. More delicately, a dysfunctional doctor was made to see early retirement due to health as a blessed release.

I was the invisible hand in these acts of self-serving mercy. Human Resources did the footwork. Cassandra said if made too public it might be tantamount to admitting the management had been in the wrong. And, as Mal Combes had endlessly quoted since I gave Nasty Ed Dorn's book of epigrams, *Yellow Lola*, 'Admission of error is a weakness of judgement if one senses beforehand that it will be seen as a weakness.' I was perfectly happy with my neo-Manichean restraint in foregoing the credit for solving intractable problems. I felt virtuous as a charity donor who remains anonymous.

But I didn't want to think about a doctor in the trust that Dean Slowey's peer review had identified as quite dangerous. I was hoping she could be dealt with externally. When Cassandra informed me that the errant had applied for maternity leave, I visited her to deliver my congratulations. But in my crash course on disciplinary protocol I learned the humane approach was sorely tested with high-paid professionals. Lawyers are employed ('Do you know how much I cost per hour?'), and little unremembered acts of kindness and love were not in your gift. Cases usually went to the bitter end when the line manager donned the metaphorical black hat. And then there were the appeals.

SAFE CONDUCT

The annual report to the Health Authorities was something of a formality. The Sibyl's feel-good factor reigned. The Powers That Be were saying, 'Don't bring us your problems, only your solutions.' The Great and Good echoed them and I gave them what was wanted, obfuscating optimistically and, accordingly, receiving their stamp of approval. I didn't mention the mess left by Harry Huggins's inaction. Or complain about inadequate resources. When asked by a member about the crisis ('failing' was a forbidden word), I said 'What crisis?' and spoke about the Big Push. Everybody was happy.

Virchow drifted into a grey area of my mind. I stopped dreaming of him. I was a serious person. The talking in my head had given up on me. MacCrone paid me a surprise visit to my cubbyhole. I took it as a sign that my seamlessness made them wonder if I still existed other than on paper. I tried to entertain him with the usual platter of ironies washed down with a digestive of what I took to be common sense, and he stopped me: 'Well done. You've balanced the books,' and smiled. Creative accounting had been assumed. My explanation of how it was achieved was so on message for the Sibyl's government that his scepticism was reinforced. True to say, the money for property deals hadn't entered the budget yet. The finance manager had concealed some underspends from the previous year. Huggins's stasis had its useful side.

MacCrone scuttled off, content that I was conforming to expectations, and, at the same time, getting around the rules of probity. His 'well done', delivered with perfunctory aplomb, was to acknowledge that I was a fellow servant of the devil. But when he looked around my converted toilet, his air of disbelief gave me a perverse pleasure. To him I resembled Mr Kurtz in the *Heart of Darkness*.

Indeed, the property venture had exceeded my highest hopes. London was a boom town for vendors. Once again luck or fate intervened. Lady Wilton of the Great and Good owned Ethical Rentals, and offered its services, waiving the fee. Health service property could not be sold, but renting suited me. I could choose tenants' clients with a health orientation. I turned down a dubious exercise centre, and experimented with a health-food cafe/shop. But when I saw their price for dandelions, I wondered about exploitation of common weeds by capitalist ecology. I was relieved when approached by the Bright Young Specialists, courtesy of Mal Combes. They wanted premises in central London for some private practice on the side. Dean Slowey suggested that I should agree on the proviso that health service referrals were treated on the National Health Service, with the clinician who sent them assisting.

The Bright Young Specialists leapt at this training initiative, seeing it as the back door to research. They needed publications to advance their reputation abroad. One of them knew the junior Mandarin whose thesis was on cost-benefit, and had divined that computerised records of case histories would lead to a study. Research on live patients *in situ* excited them. It was on the crest of advanced epidemiological thinking, and would attract funding, not only from the usual suspects (the drugs, tobacco and sugar industries). The Medical Research Council was now keen on research in the real world.

The Mandarins were taken by the training and cost-benefit dimension. Elective treatments being withdrawn from costly hospitals pleased the Health Authorities. Local clinicians saw it as a chance to hone their skills, impress their patients, and improve their prospects of some private practice. Everybody was pleased except the Eminents. They liked to swan around with the hospital Consultants. But times were changing, and opportunities needed to be seized. Squatters had taken over the basement in the disused hospital in Soho. Social services wanted to make it into a centre for homeless people. The Eminents suggested a health dimension with Murdock Gow, the youngest Eminent, as the lead. Money would come from charities, supplemented by London Council, which was keen to clean up the city. As the trust owned the site, I would be the wren riding the Eminents' eagle. They hadn't thought of that.

The feel-good factor did not exclude a one per cent budget cut for trusts. Reductions in services were easier to understand and reward. Electoral rolls ruled their interest, and numbers spoke louder than ideas. When the Mandarins raised cost-benefit considerations, the Powers That Be, the cabinet ministers, turned a deaf ear, preferring to listen to public-spirited millionaires. Their advice was to loosen up employment law, regulate trade unions, deregulate banks, and shrink public services. Education, health and social services were seen as a burden on tax payers (the only society the Sibyl believed in). The aim was to standardise them at the lowest common denominator. Expectations had to be reduced to bring more people into private insurance. In effect all public services were failing. They needed to be dismantled to make them more efficient.

'Yes, it's everyone for himself,' Mal Combes said. 'Draw water from the well, build your sandcastles. But know, Poet, that you're working in an oasis which is likely to become a mirage. The population isn't getting any younger. And the government, to prevent the old becoming a burden on the state, will bring in euthanasia. Don't get carried away.' However, that summer a ferry load of merry nurses and secretaries returning from Calais, laden with wine and French clothes, were singing 'Trust and Obey'. Everybody was into irony and it was a good time for it. But I allowed myself to get carried away. It gave me pleasure to know there was such a thing as real fun, and it was part of their job.

VI

GETTING THINGS UNDONE

'Big ideas are the enemy of little ideas.'

—Brecht

VIRCHOW DOUBTS

MY DETERMINATION TO GET THINGS DONE WAS occasionally weakened by doubts about the larger idea. When things seemed to be going well, I was most vulnerable. Something inconsequential caught my eye, and second thoughts nagged.

While on my clinic rounds I picked up a *Reader's Digest* in a waiting room, and read that elephants died of starvation once they lost their third set of teeth. I laughed. Jo Manders would fit the edentulous elephants with false teeth. The funding would be from the ivory trade (an unwise investment – it's doubtful that aged elephants could reproduce). I thought of the consequences of Jo's intervention. It would radically change jungle life. Ever increasing herds of giant pachyderms eating their way through the undergrowth would reduce the vegetation that nourishes the roots of trees. And so the jungle forest would thin down, and gradually return to marsh or desert. The elephants would starve to death anyway.

I mulled over Virchow's long-term consequences. A health-driven mankind would fare no better than the elephants. The body's wear and tear is not a disease to be cured. Once the bone is eroded from normal usage, tooth loss and loss of appetite would be inevitable. Virchow must ultimately fail. Nobody is going to live forever, or if they do their fate will be that of Swift's Struldbrugs (*Gulliver's Travels*), to fade and wither into perpetual Alzheimer's.

Mal Combes's 'Forget about the big ideas… the devil is in the detail' began to seem less small-minded. I knew from my childhood that there were big questions that made people sit up and put on their best ideas. In the open family forum, that came with a hearth to savour the smell of burning wood and a fire to warm the hands; we were on the edge of our seats. My rawest infant memory was in the winter of the big freeze in 1947. Post-war Europe was in shreds, and the weather added to its woes. Due to fuel shortages, in the subsequent general election the Attlee government lost the majority that swept in the welfare state. It survived, just.

The amplitude of my father's ideas made me forget my chilblains. The end of civilisation as we know it was the burning issue. But my mother was impatient with his despair at the scramble for a new world order. 'The leaders should be put in a field and made to fight it out themselves.' Single-handed combat caught my fancy. I could understand that, and that peace and quiet is what most people want.

As I grew up I learnt from her to be suspicious of the big ideas that can't be felt or smelt. Sometimes they are simple like

Christianity and Marxism. At odds with one another despite much in common. Treat everybody as you would yourself. Share and share alike. What fragrance! Then they become too big and lose touch. The big ideas come with crushing responsibilities. History is steam-rollered with their bloody consequences. Who wants to be Napoleon, Stalin, Hitler or Winston Churchill, except madmen? Yet they are the world historical figures. Social reformers who think small and act prudently, like Pierre Waldeck-Rousseau and William Morris are remembered only as an afterthought, usually kindly, if reminded by a street sign or Pre-Raphaelite wallpaper.

However, Waldeck-Rousseau as *premier ministre* modernised France. Not only did he recognise workers rights by legalising trade unions in 1884 (thirteen years after Britain), but at the turn of the century he sorted out the Dreyfus scandal by censoring the army, and with *Laïcité* separated the church from the state (it became law in 1905 after his premature death). All done with a minimum of fuss in a deeply divided nation. And William Morris, by way of Robert Owen, brought Anarchism down to earth with the Cooperative Movement, which still thrives in quiet corners of the globe. Little ideas do their work purely and simply. They function and don't expect to be remembered for it.

The talking in my head wondered about the simple. It's easier to think big and act small than to think small and act big. It's easier to kill than prevent a killing. The talking was now in full rant. Making health and well-being an absolute at all costs is to damn small important matters such as moral justice, high culture and the freedom to live dangerously.

I said to the talking, 'silence seduces', borrowing René Char's shut-up. There was consolation in thinking Virchow was really a little idea. Although maybe that's why Bismarck's Germany didn't take it seriously, despite implications far greater than the Iron Chancellor's Empire-building. The consequences of Virchow are big enough to boost moral concerns rather than override them, and reconcile German Idealism and Marxist materialism. Assuming, as Descartes did, that the body's well-being is good for the immortal soul *and* the state of the world.

JUDGE-PENITENT

Whatever my grandiose ideas around Virchow, getting things done was overtaken by things I had to undo. I had my hands full with disciplinary cases. Despite Dick Cross's winnowing of them, a dozen were outstanding. There were three main categories. The backlog from Harry Huggins, those arising from peer review (mostly in other trusts), and cases I had initiated myself. In Harry, or peer review-associated, hearings a line manager conducted the case. I could be called to give evidence, but mostly I just sat in as an observer.

Sometimes it was like eavesdropping on a confessional box. Other times it was a formal procedure going through its paces, the outcome preordained. But when I saw a presumed errant made utterly miserable, a tear suppressed or visible signs of self-anger, I did not hide my face behind the proffered hanky, or gesture of sympathy. I betrayed emotion which was contrary to the process. But I found being cruel to the particular to be kind to the general was ugly, almost like shooting deserters in a civil war (something my father's generation had to deal with). That it was a necessary evil didn't make it any less of one, I thought.

It was only a difference in kind from your victim's. Of course all justice is rough and, when holding back my feelings proved impossible, I bit my lip, and pretended I had got something caught in my eye. It was pathetic. Afterwards when I spoke to Cassandra she said only the offer of the hanky had been noticed.

In cases I had initiated, I was the judge and jury. A sense of responsibility hardened me. I was cast iron. But not above using emotion to get a response when the case was getting nowhere. I thought it wouldn't be necessary when the offence could be deemed criminal. That is, when the suffering of others was greater than that of the perpetrator. But in manipulating things through a display of emotion I was my mother's son. It wasn't coldly calculated. But I knew that by touching the heartstrings in a hopeless case you could get unexpected about-turns, a confession or an eleventh-hour resignation. Once, in the relief of the moment, I offered a written reference. I reassured an unhappy Cassandra that it would be undated, and coded. Only a prospective employer who was careless would not ring me up.

When the greater good obliged me to go to the wire and fire someone for reasons that were not cut and dried, I was not unknown to withhold information that might be considered extenuating circumstances. It was for the other side to raise it, I said. When Dick Cross was present he usually did. But he left cases with professional associations to their own union representative. And since the extenuating circumstances were, more often than not, personal, pleading them was professionally embarrassing for doctors and dentists, and avoided. Cycling along the Grand Union towpaths reminded me that the judge-penitent in Camus' *La Chute* accused himself of enjoying lying by omission so much that he always arranged to have something to hide. He wasn't bothered by his duplicity, until the famous cry from the canal woke his conscience. I turned off my Walkman, but I didn't hear the voice of my victims.

Disciplinary hearings in theory are about truth-telling and exposure. In practice they are about concealment and lies of omission. The talking in my head was relentless. I was becoming so self-critical that Cassandra after one hearing joked that she thought I was going to dismiss myself. Indeed the babble in my head was akin to a cornered scholastic trying to make sense of the Inquisition. I could control myself, but not the consequences. Still, I didn't want to become a dead-bat sentimentalist, like Ivan in Dostoyevsky's *The Brothers Karamazov,* and lose faith because I couldn't face the imagined tears of the ex-employee's children.

Cassandra advised me to stick to a verifiable fact directly related to the offence. 'It may not be the most serious one, but it should be enough to get a result.' 'So ideas don't matter then,' I flared. 'You mean opinions,' she dared. But Montaigne, the most sensible of thinkers, helped me to get a grip on myself. 'We reason rashly and at random because our judgements – like ourselves – have in them a large element of chance.' But I wasn't leaving everything to chance. I instigated a ledger for the administration to log untoward incidents, and called it the Moby Book. I can't remember why but it stuck. A meticulous recording of signal events for a potential disciplinary action was a small idea. If it materialised, I had the body of evidence for what needed to be done, and it wouldn't involve soul searching. I was readying myself for the black-hat moment and when I pronounced the final word it would be as a functionary, not God.

I gave myself a good talking to, made a mantra of the one idea I was sure of, and recited it to myself to banish doubt. *Something had to be done to get people to do their job properly.* By clinging to this basic aspiration I found I could function without tormenting myself. I did what I had to and got on with what was next. Maintaining a dumb-focus with the small idea, helped to suppress righteous anger, and pointless sympathy, perishing thoughts that were not directly related to the task at hand. 'The custom and practice of ordinary life bears us along,' says Montaigne, who was a judge-penitent.

However the severity of the fact could be softened once it was put in context. The Moby Book could serve as a preventive. Once an incident was logged the administrator had a quiet word with the main protagonist. More often than not there was a reasonable explanation. For instance, when a log in the Moby Book related to something not done, Cassandra looked up the employee's job description to see if the underperformance could be due to a mutual misunderstanding of duties. Sometimes the job description merely needed changing so expectations were made clear. Negotiating this either brought a new lease of life, or the employee resigned.

When there was trouble brewing I took to visiting the clinic informally for a casual chat with the potential errant. For example, internal complaints had reached the Moby Book that patients were claiming a certain clinician was hopelessly ill-organised. There was merit in starting with the lowest common denominator of competence. Noting the tea-and-coffee arrangements could be instructive. Percolating machines needing coffee beans to be ground, or the sending of staff out to queue for drinks, indicated questionable priorities.

'Haven't you got an electric kettle?' I asked. 'I've brought my teabag.' Raising an issue that was seen as a small matter didn't challenge others' *amour propre* and lightly made a pertinent point.

'But we have to go out for milk.'

'Powdered is fine for me.'

Mutual amusement became part of the process. Still the confrontation acted as a model and point of reference for larger considerations which would have to be tackled. As I didn't know where to begin, the visits fizzled out.

Chronic entrants in the Moby Book were often the result of impasses that others had failed to breach. If they were problems in interpersonal relations I left it to Human Resources. There was the case of a certain Dr Marcos. His recurrent entries related to staff infighting, and his behaviour had become increasingly misanthropic. Nobody wanted to work with him. And patients became frightened when nurses burst into tears.

Cassandra talked to him, but Dr Marcos was adamant that he was only upholding standards: 'I'm a training resource, a free gift to further education.' 'Greeks,' she said, 'they're so logical you can't contradict them. I was exhausted into agreeing with him.'

I said, 'If a patient complains, no matter how minor, I'll give him a warning. After that he will have to watch himself.'

'And you'll have to watch yourself. Beware of Greeks bearing gifts.'

'He's my Trojan Horse, you mean.'

Cassandra laughed, 'No, Marcos is a rocking horse.'

'Straw by straw the bird builds its nest' was the heading of my first newsletter for staff. I rejected just in time the French proverb 'each nail follows the next' when Mal Combes pointed out that

I wasn't working on a coffin. I floated, 'the nailing I had in mind was more on hands,' and his speech melody was not harmonious to me: 'Ah, it's your own funeral.'

We were not on the same wavelength. When I proposed instead 'doctor heal thyself', to 'empower them', he gave me an irritated look. Quoting from the Bible was the last straw. Although I paid heed to him and settled for 'singing from the same hymn sheet' I didn't hear from him for several months.

Indeed, I had Mal Combes withdrawal symptoms. But I avoided passing his garden, or showing off to Nasty that I had read Proust (most of it anyway, in my days of Ordinary Madness). And so, when he rang me ('Poet, I have something I want you to do'), it lifted my spirits. But, before responding, I first mentioned the coffin exchange and he recalled, 'You were overestimating your poor staff's cultural references so much that I wanted to scream. Plus, at the time I had enough trouble on my hands dealing with the senior Consultants over the damn training and development idea that Dean Slowey put you up to.'

LOST SHEEP IN WHITE COATS

Mal Combes's request gave me something to do, other than trying to mend what wasn't broken. In a large organisation there is always an engine that keeps it turning over. The day-to-day running was encrusted with old girls proud of their slow but sure administration. These office clerks were the backbone of the city hall that once ran health and social services. Their leading light was Lucenda Lucas, the keeper of the Moby Book. Her assistants were mostly young women from the provinces, glad to be living in the capital. Mrs Lucas would take them under her wing, and crabbed age and youth worked like a madrigal together.

Finance management was in the hands of exiled Kenyan Asians, led by my old friend, Rami Bashir (whose work ethic was what allowed him eight hours of sleep a night). He had tricks up his sleeve that were borderline legal. The last-minute viring of under-spends to an over-spend budget to avoid the excesses disappearing back into the departmental coffers was only the half of it. The safety net for his fiscal trapeze act was a boyish enthusiasm that masked cold calculations. He was a step ahead of even the Mandarins' accountants.

Mal Combes wanted me 'to provide a home for the rehabilitation of professionals. The Medical Council are looking for one, and you already know the ropes.' My previous experience was in my freelance days of Ordinary Madness. Mal Combes had been researching dentists struck off the register for drug abuse. The prevailing view at the Medical Council was that professionals caught sniffing the ether ought to be struck off the register for life. Mal Combes had challenged that, and obtained money from the Mandarins, claiming it was from their 'eco-pot' for recycling wastage.

I was to find them work experience around and about McCall and Manders's Good Spit project. Mal Combes dubbed it grandparenting, even though I was much younger than most of my charges. When they presented themselves wearing three-piece suits I groomed them to relax into casual clothes. I got them to assist Jo Manders in making dentures for the centenarians. She nicknamed them the Lazaruses. Their pale undernourished appearance made them look as though they had been recently dug up. 'Where came ye, pallid wanderers,' I sighed, as they tried to be useful. Alas, Jo had no time for, or patience with, them, and, one by one, they disappeared. I never knew what happened to them.

This time the Medical Council took a hard line against Mal Combes's idea on the grounds that with the emergence of HIV from dirty needles, ex-drug addicts were a risk to patients. He responded that with routine cross-infection procedures the chances of transmission should be nil. They ceded ungraciously under pressure from the Mandarins, who, Mal Combes told me, believed the Medical Council might want to issue sterner diktats on clinical hygiene.

The new wave of drug errants were not much better than the Lazaruses. Baudelaire, who knew about opiates, might have been describing them when he spoke of: 'artificial men activated by strange springs.' There were four, all doctors and male. I re-christened them the Bartlebys, after the reluctant scrivener in Melville's short story. Like him, they would have preferred not to be there. They held up the walls of my cubbyhole of an office and so, when I entered, it was as though someone had planted cardboard cut-outs there. Stiff and tongue-tied, they carried white coats under their arms. I lightened the atmosphere by telling the story about the previous wave and Jo's Good Spit project. That encouraged them to speak not merely when spoken to. I laughed off the idea of grandparenting, saying my role would be more peer pressure. 'We are all professionals.'

I took them around the wards and clinics, introducing them as doctors from elsewhere. They followed me like lost sheep. As the day wore on I realised their existential embarrassment at their situation was not dissimilar to mine. And, like me, it made them verbal float, and say things they didn't quite mean.

One Bartleby talked himself up extravagantly. Another laughed too loudly, making jokes at his own expense. The remaining two spoke as though they were reciting from a manual of how to make a good impression in a bad situation. I needed clues to find them suitable placements for their development, but I was getting nowhere. I remembered Count Alfieri's advice to diplomats, 'pay attention to even the most foolish remark as frequently it's a cover for what is not being said. You learn more from what is withheld.' Their speech melodies were atonal, but there was nothing withheld in their body language. It spoke eloquently. These were men desperate to right their lives, but doubting themselves.

The Bartlebys were employed as care assistants to doctors on the wards. They had to have a proper job, Dick Cross rightly said. At our weekly meeting over tea and biscuits, the braggart said that they would have preferred to be considered voluntary workers and not paid. 'But it means you have a real job,' I said, 'and that's a first step,' adding, as I poured the tea, 'It's not uncommon for overseas graduates seeking permits to practise in England to take work in hospitals in modest jobs.'

In dealing with my Bartlebys, I applied Theodore Roosevelt's dictum, 'speak softly and carry a big stick.' I was nice and nasty as required. While pooh-poohing any signs of self-abasement or self-pity, I pulled up sharp self-aggrandisement, and ingratiating clichés. A particular defect of someone coming out of a brain-compromising experience is repeating oneself. I brought this to their attention by playing back a recording I made of a conversation. My 'there we go again', induced nervous laughter. But it was a bad mistake. What amounted to a bugging device reduced their confidence in me. I learned to exercise patience in order to keep my temperament in rein. I was testing myself too. My low tolerance threshold at meetings needed to be addressed.

The Bartlebys were being reconditioned. It was like secondary socialisation in a crèche, but with the grown-ups on the high chairs. I tried to be like a child watching adults in his place, and the reversal of roles was instructive. Once my charges got over their sense of humiliation, anger with themselves surfaced. They had not only one another to vent it on, they had me. Their anger pleased me. Pride was returning. And they were angry with their past selves. They were able to look back.

I sensed they were on the mend when they began to speak about their work as care assistants, exchanging jokes on the immediate reality, and questioning the system. This did their confidence, and mine in them, a world of good. And I learned something. Once you go beyond self-deception, or fear of failing again, even though you're not where you want to be, dignity is restored. I risked losing them by confiding my feeling of 'getting away with things' and the sense of embarrassment that dogged my life. But not at all. It was an experience they all had lived in their addict days.

Progress mutually recognised, I stopped thinking of them as the Bartlebys. They became colleagues who worked well together, a form of friendship that I think is underestimated. We wrote a charter for care assistants together, which I was able to use to start a peer review group. After six months I wrote a report on each, suggesting the next steps in their rehabilitation. Shortly afterwards they were taken off my hands. Some years later I asked Mal Combes what happened to them. Only the self-mocker regained his registration with the Medical Council.

The braggart had disappeared before the exams, and was said to be working without a permit in South Africa. But the two who seemed to speak from a crib surprised me. I revised my view on Count Alfieri's advice. What was unspoken was that they had lost taste for the profession that had led them to this unpretty pass. One retrained as a vet, the other as a medical librarian. I thought that I was the redemption and the light. But their destiny was to be found sitting in their own minds, not mine. The vet had a problem with people, and the librarian loved books.

I kept the ex-Bartlebys at the back of my head when dealing with staff who made the Moby Book. I was merely a vessel, a *lacrimatoire*, to pour their tears into to become relics. My modus operandi changed. I maintained a decent distance between myself and the potential errants, and so necessary reproofs weren't too personal. It was up to them if they were up to it. This took the weight of moralising off my conscience. I listened and learned. What was happening existed in a sphere beyond me. I was merely giving it a wave, waving it on.

Nevertheless, I wrote a verse, 'I Am a Teapot', and pinned it behind my desk:

> Please feel free to pour out.
> I am a container,
> capacity limit-
> ed by side and bottom,
> but with an open top
> to drain off overflows,
> and a sponge reservoir
> underneath to sop up.
> Be mother or whoever.

Thus the door was open like Jean Renoir's film set. Anyone could walk in to change the shooting script. I thought of putting the last words of *The Rules of the Game* on my noticeboard: 'Everybody has their reasons'. I changed my mind. What might walk in my door could be more reasonable than I thought, and prove unmanageable.

LOSING FRIENDS

Creeping privatisation came to see me in a Savile Row suit. He was one of the business consultants involved in the feasibility study for independent trusts. Like the PR policeman who came to appease me after I had been declared dead by default, his main interest was in property. 'Your trust must be worth millions,' he said. 'No,' I replied, 'We rent it.' He got my answer the wrong way round, thinking we paid rent rather than collected it, and lost interest. Then he went on to talk about Harley Street becoming an outpost of Guy's Hospital. Or was it other way round? His tautology cheered me up. The audit hadn't reached the serious stage.

Mrs Sibyl's feel-good campaign failed to produce the desired effect. People weren't fooled by her Leibnizian *optimisme*. They knew that Mrs Sibyl wanted them to feel good about themselves in order to feel good about herself. She castigated a despondent population for being unpatriotic. Union Jack underwear was worn over trousers by punks groaning:

> God save the queen.
> She ain't no human being.

There's no future
in England's dreaming.
No future, no future
for you or me.

Her huff was just a last puff. Boadicea had overreached herself, and was losing battles. Her three 'No's to a promising peace process to end the war in Ireland was in effect a last stand. She was living in a power bubble, which would grow until it burst. Her party already had lined up a stalking horse, not so much to challenge her, but as a warning. Behind the 'also ran' the favourites were champing at the bit. In short, the Elders were preparing to pay a visit to the bunker to tell her the time was propitious to step down.

The hysterical/historical moment she had unleashed, when anything could happen, was over, and it was only a matter of time before there was a regime change, and the thrice-defeated opposition stood in the wings with a brushed up image. Formerly the workingman's party, it was now the party of refracted public opinion. Pride in its socialist past had been replaced by being all things to all men (and women), and the tabloid press. The class struggle was over. 'We're all middle class now and proud of it.' Mrs Sibyl was silently acknowledged.

Trade unions were never the same since the defeat of the miners' strike. Membership had halved since the seventies. Their financial support was almost an embarrassment to the New Brooms. Increased contributions from business would make them more electable. Capital and labour could be reconciled by mutual investment. Yet cynics said that the New Broom was made up of the bits and pieces of the old broom. They were right in one essential. The New Broom promised to restore equilibrium to the Established Order. Not as a regressive sweep, of course. It would be modernised by the Hoover of Public Relations.

The Eminents were not unhappy, and the Great and Good were making new friends. The Mandarins heaved a sigh of relief. The turbulence of the last decade had been bad for their digestion. Now they could hope to resume their rightful place at the feast. Then the unexpected happened. Mrs Sibyl resigned. It was whispered for health reasons. And the quietest of her young men, Little John, took over. He was in personality and character a perfect antidote to the Sibyl, talking of 'back to basics'. Nostalgia for the future spoke to Middle England. 'Fifty years from now Britain will still be a country of long shadows on the cricket field, warm beer, invisible leafy suburbs, dog lovers and pool fillers.' His personal popularity swept away the New Broom. When he won the election, he retained the Sibyl's less controversial policies. But learning from her mistakes, he realised that without the resurgent Established Order behind him, his government wouldn't survive. The New Broom's Hoover was safe in his hands.

Mal Combes said, 'It was just a change in scenery. It would take ages for the Established Order to get themselves together. And with the pressure off the Mandarins, they would not be incurious as to the cost-benefits of your schemes. You should renew "putting proven solutions into practice". It's a project that could tap into private/public partnerships. Not least with the pharmaceutical industry. Little John prides himself in being non-ideological, and open to the practical. Your ideas will be seen as prudent and uncontroversial. His people will run with them.'

I had my doubts, but I contacted Dean Slowey. His retirement beckoned, and he recommended I talk to Angus Cook, one of my Bright Young Specialists ('He has a foot in every camp, including the Eminents'). He had dentists in London still using silver nitrate, a discredited material, identified. The Health Authority sent them the standard letter that had been devised for outmoders, signed by Angus. A few doctors in inner London were still prescribing antibiotics to children that caused teeth to go black. Sales reps were encouraged to visit these practices to furnish them with free samples of safe alternatives.

I couldn't claim importance to humanity, à la Virchow, only importance to the immediate situation. My aim was simply to do something about what is obvious to anyone who has been mistreated by a medical man. I doodled a cartoon of Boadicea being tripped up by a leprechaun dressed in nineteenth-century drainpipes and frockcoat. The caption read 'Gotcha!' (a tabloid headline from when the Sibyl sank a ship of Argentinean conscripts in the battle for the Malvinas). I pinned it on the wall behind my desk in the cubbyhole with Virchow's law under it in bold capitals. When asked what it meant, I floated, 'It's a secular prayer. You've just got to believe it.'

Weary of living on my wits, I let the trust get on with itself, and made a last trip down to see Edna Gray. She too was retiring, and feeling low. Her studies of average work-output included the death rate in general practices. The results had been ignored during Mrs Sibyl's feel-good period. Since then she had observed significant statistical differences between hospitals in heart-surgery deaths, particularly in children, and even her friend the Dean had failed to interest Consultant groups, let alone the Department of Health. She was right about the scandals to come, but died of leukaemia before she could bemoan the failure to prevent them.

I felt the human warmth in her farewell as a dying fall. And on the train to London I was thoughtful. Once Dean Slowey retired, I would have no friends, except Mal Combes, and he would make me more enemies. My dumb-focus hardened. I told myself, 'Blinkers are necessary to keep going. Actions speak. Talk does not act.'

ALL SWINGING TOGETHER

The pity about luck is it runs out. Little John's path was paved with stumbling blocks thrown up by a steep recession (which Mrs Sibyl must have seen coming, biting the bullet by joining the European Exchange Rate a month before she resigned). His 'back to basics' became backs to the wall. On Black Wednesday (16 September 1992) an attempt to save sterling from devaluation failed miserably. Billions of the national reserves disappeared into the stock market. The New Broom flayed around, but didn't force a general election. Little John did what he could, which wasn't much. But the peace process in Ireland benefited as a distraction.

As the Established Order reordered, the culture of corporateness reasserted itself. The hymn sheet now was the 'Eton Boating Song'. My mother was right. Everybody knew their place and the place of others. But I evaded mine and others sensed that I didn't recognise theirs. The Eminent Persons Group, their iron bottoms newly polished, were firmly in the driving seat. My dumb-focus pragmatism was seen as getting ahead of myself. The ex-scapegoat needed to be reined in.

The reason for the corporate spirit was not just power politics. It had deep indigenous roots. I remember being told about the farm labourers who emigrated to England in the 1950s to work on building sites. Accustomed to hard work, the navvies redoubled their efforts to counter the prejudice that the Irish are lazy. Soon enough they were taken aside by the English workers and told that the more you do the less overtime time we'll get.

At a professional level, the difference was in degree rather than kind. I thought honest industry was the prime Protestant virtue. And that, if I worked my hob-nailed boots off in England, it would be enough to gain approval. But the approbation, and a job for life, was for working the way everybody else did. This especially applied to change. Not that change wasn't accepted as inevitable, but it had to take place at a rate that brought the reluctant rump along with it. Nobody was to be left behind. That slowed things down to a mutually agreeable pace. By the time change was negotiated into progress, the original impulse might have lost its spontaneity, but it was solidly entrenched. The Established Order was backed by the weight of numbers and the country advanced in solid plods.

FOR THE BIRDS

I could hear Max Madison say, 'It's an excellent idea, but it lacks arse. It's for the birds.' In his English conservative way he believed ideas must come directly from what went before. They had to be in keeping with the consensual lurch. Thus the Established Order 'continues because it had begun'. Nevertheless, Britain has a glorious history of lone inventors who changed the world, from Roger Bacon to Alexander Graham Bell, Charles Babbage, John Logie Baird... These hummingbirds of invention appear from nowhere (or Scotland), zigzagging to earth to peck up the grains to make their own manna. Their light and airy flits and purposeful darts could achieve more in a day than the corporate flocks in a year of waiting for the grain to grow and be cropped.

The Great and Good, as high-flyers, ought to admire the hummingbirds' capacity to soar. Indeed, once upon a time, they would have been their patrons. But the twentieth century's politicisation of science through a barrage of regulations has made them wary of sharing their airspace. The Powers That Be might shoot them down by mistake. They find it prudent to keep their feet on a secure launching pad, an aircraft carrier like their Eminent Persons Group. The Established Order huddles together on deck, doing the groundwork with endless planning committees, and sub-groups. Cumbersome and gravid as Howard Hughes's jumbo aircraft, the *Spruce Goose*, which on its one and only flight, bumped along just above the surface, only to subside under its own weight back on to the runway.

I was only a chick hummingbird, my contrivances scarcely hatched. But I was made to suffer for it by the Eminents. 'You're your own worst enemy,' Dame Brenda said to me when I expressed impatience at yet another hoop to jump through to get something off the ground. But I listened to the old fox Stanley O. Kay. 'You flighty ones have only yourselves to blame. You don't think about what's already there, the gains made against the grain over the years. There is a time for doing and a time to refrain...' And he was right. As the recession pinched, the Mandarins told the Health Authorities to do nothing drastic. Just keep things going as before.

My bird had been grounded since I ceased to be freelance and took to management territory. Although I sometimes got carried away, forgetting my wings had been clipped, I had to lower my sights, raise my chicken-flap, and run with the Established Order, one short step at a time. A job to be done became my poor-man's credo and not wasting my time, my catechism. And so I was left to my own devices, and did nothing except appear busy. That was easy. The Health Authority or the Mandarins rarely contacted me. Mal Combes had given up on me again. But I hadn't quite given up on myself. Maybe I'll serve someone's purpose again, I said to myself, not too convinced. Mrs Sibyl had run out of fire, Little John of steam, but the diesel-driven New Broom to come might well regard me as lead, and have me removed. Meanwhile, 'In the battle between oneself and the world, support the world,' Kafka wrote to a fellow functionary in health insurance. The best way to avoid the chop is to keep your head down.

THE NIGHT OF THE KNOCKING

Alone in my Panopticon prison tower (sight-unseen, but appearing to see all), I didn't need to keep my head down. However, beyond my vantage point I could hear the murmur of continuous conversation, and I had to block it out to listen to what was sitting on my mind. 'As long as you don't know what is going on everything is all right.'

As my mother's son I knew it was a time for masterful inaction. I was in a 'didn't' phase. This was made easier as the Ground Forces preferred not to trouble me. My social contacts were limited to people at work that I couldn't avoid. At home my solipsism was as absolute as Claude Brunet's *Pensée Solitaire*.

Reality was all in the mind. During evenings I opened a bottle of wine, lit my pipe and wrote down anything that came into my head. 'If a drop of wine dribbles down the bottle, you must lick it off.' Sentences of fourteen words appeared to write themselves.

Rilke came to mind. He dreamed of a day when at his command, 'words, glorious words, appear on the page, that are not my own. One word upon another, given meaning like a cloud that breaks into rain.' But I plumped for a Berkeleyan explanation for these word sonnets. George Berkeley had been the Bishop of Cloyne. The town has a hump bridge and, as a boy being driven over it, it invariably gave me a jolt. I was convinced it was the ghost of the first philosopher of solipsism going bump. And now I was bumping along, bringing my own world into existence.

As night fell the talking in my head was interrupted by a sonic disturbance, a persistent knocking sound. It was like a door with a loose lock rattling in a storm. Yet the door was securely fitted, and there was no wind. I closed the windows, turned off electrical appliances, including the lights. Now the knocking was counter-pointed by the sound of an insistent internal drip. But all the taps were firmly sealed. I recorded the double-stopping on my portable Dictaphone for Dr Jack, my psychologist friend. If I spoke to him about my sleep complex and fear of outside interference it would be evidence. But nothing registered on the tape.

Insomnia is a time for second thoughts. Although Berkeley didn't believe in the objective world – you make it all up by yourself – its continued existence depended on someone being there to observe what is essentially you. 'The material world is an "idea" that only exists when a mind discovers it. *To be is to be perceived.'* I asked myself if there was someone looking through the keyhole, and answered the door. But there was nobody there. Maybe it was reality trying to get in to tell me not to be mad: it had a life of its own and to recreate it out of my head would be to get it wrong.

When I returned to bed the drip's splashes had become more emphatic, disturbing me more than the timid knocks. I would have done anything to hear nothing. Stuffing my ears with cotton wool, I thought of Vincent Van Gogh, and of when I attended the Rice Festival corrida in Arles. I watched as the sword stuck on the third attempt between the heaving withers of a bull, drooling blood. A cart dragged off the carcass as the matador was awarded an ear, which he dedicated to a woman in the tribune who threw it back.

Now the drip beat seemed to be conducting the subliminal hum of the city. Traffic differentiated itself into the stops and starts of cars, the squeal of brakes and the occasional horn. The details of a world in the small hours were coming alive. And yet, according to Berkeley, the facts under description were events happening in my head, and only existed because I was perceived perceiving it.

A security alarm went off in the house opposite. No lights came on. The house was vacant. For almost an hour, the talking in my head was drowned out. Maybe the alarm was my Berkeleyan defence to quell thoughts I would prefer not to entertain. Wallace Stevens, the most Berkeleyan of poets, thought, 'It is a violence from within that protects us from the violence without. The imagination presses back against the pressure of reality.' But it was the 'violence without' that was protecting me from the 'violence within'. When the alarm turned itself off as suddenly as it had begun, the rattling at the door came back as a light unassuming knock, polite as a wake-up call in a family hotel.

The talking in my head chided me: 'It's time to take the berk out of your Berkeleyism. The good bishop was an empiricist, who at heart wanted an imaginary existence in the eyes of others, and speculated so it could be reciprocated. David Hume took him up and carried his pure ideas as far as they could go. But Hume changed his mind at the eleventh hour. He knew that no matter what you think, things won't work out as you imagined. The sun will rise tomorrow, with or without you.'

The first shaft of daylight entered the room. Not a bright new dawn for early morning eyes that hadn't slept a wink. But it was a start. I walked to work by the longest way round, fortified with good intentions. Managers may be the prime mover but secondary considerations mean that you get things done, or not, as circumstances present themselves.

DAWN

Still, my mind was racing like a loose horse in the Grand National. I jumped the fences on my own. I wouldn't interfere with the other runners. My leading position would only fool the visually challenged, and those ignorant of the rules.

But I was pulled up by a Tube station under reconstruction. I noticed that the navvies were all black. They had changed colour, apparently overnight. Where were the Irish? Returning to Ireland to buy the farms their fathers rented? Or maybe it was the dirty conditions. They were like miners coming up from the pits. Black but still Irish... I was drifting. The dandelion fluff and feathers of moulting geese in St James's Park were flying around in the wind. I could chase and gather them into brown paper bags. If I could find one. Everything was plastic now.

The white-haired Rasta with the wooden cross was up early, walking the streets of Notting Hill, crying out as usual in a gentle voice, 'You have stolen my pain. You have stolen my death.' I smiled at him and he blessed me. Life is one-way. The body is for others and the mind is for yourself. And yet they are all of a piece. Descartes dissected his body with his mind, and died choking on a question-mark, crying out for an emetic, wine mixed with tobacco.

Passing Lord's Cricket Ground I remembered my dead-bat days as a boy. I only made runs when a ball from a fast bowler ricocheted off an edge. I was difficult to get out, playing for time, or light, depending on weather conditions. I don't know how many fellow batsmen I had run out by not moving when they waved their bat. The look on their faces told me I wasn't destined to be loved. Life is a team game.

I never arrived at work so early, and was surprised to find a cleaner in my cubbyhole.

'I didn't know anybody bothered to clean my office.'

She said, 'No, I just make sure your mess is in order. I'd open your windows if you had any.' She gave me a motherly smile. I felt like an infant. We talked about Galicia in the north-west of Spain (where my mother's paternal grandfather was said to have come from). Her older children were at school there. One was to start studying medicine next year. When they were little they went to the Spanish primary in Notting Hill Gate, and so they were bilingual. 'This should serve them well when we all go to America,' she said. 'Especially the Spanish.' The world was enlarged for me.

I didn't lock the door to smoke my pipe. It would be an hour or so before staff began to arrive. I reviewed my working life in tranquillity. I was lucky to have a job that I could talk to. Most wage slaves are just talked at, and can only answer by doing what they're told. Though I sometimes envied the clarity of that. You've nothing to lose, except your chains.

However, paid work was a presence in my life that called for more than a *Pensée Solitaire*. Last night's knocking was a solipsist's waking dream. The disturbances all happened in my head, but there was no knock-on effect: the world and me carried on as before. I could get on with my job. Nevertheless, I needed to take stock or I would disappear up my own air. The object of my work, getting things done, was best achieved by maintaining a dumb-focus. However, the flip side of the coin of pragmatism is reflection, and it complicates one's effectiveness. For instance, I might have thought that I was doing the right thing by quoting Virchow (or my simplification of him) but it opened me up to interrogation, not least by myself. Indeed, I questioned my job all the time, and it rarely answered the ones I asked. That led to silences. We didn't want to talk to one another. These standoffs were interrupted by the talking in my head with doubts and fears. And I clamoured to cry out to my job, 'speak to me'. I was waiting for an outburst. I wanted to be judged now, favourably or otherwise. Even a verdict that amounted to a kick in the teeth would be welcome. I wanted my job to answer back. And all I got was the great 'Nope' out there.

People say, 'It's only a job.' But work is a microcosm of our communion with what Beckett called the Great Ineffables ('eff them'): death, God, (im)mortality, human love, happiness, grief, and pain. If the job is refusing to speak to you, giving you a blank stare, there is every reason for despair. 'Mixing our labour with others,' according to Georges Bataille, 'is a form of communion more hostile and powerful than any other.' He sees the silent void opening into an abyss that beckons us to the Great Unknown. I didn't regard that as part of my job description. But a life's work does raise ontological questions. It throws us back to where we came from, and what we make of our lives.

It's not only a job, I thought. Work is a metaphorical hair-extension, but living is a bald business.

THE SLUMMING STRATEGY

This whirlwind of thought sucked me up, and I had nothing to hold on to. Outer space beckoned. But my survival instinct opened its parachute. I floated down and hit the ground still running, and skidded into action. I was in overdrive, and my breathlessness came with a 'curious puffing' like *le pauvre* in the Wallace Stevens poem 'The Plot Against the Giant'. But I was whispering 'gutturals' rather than 'heavenly labials'. I was undoing my ideas. When the Ground Forces saw me coming they hid in a doorway, the Upper Echelons pulled up short to let me pass and, if I knocked into an Eminent or a Great and Good, their respective abruptness and politeness made for an exchange short and sweet as a donkey's tail. Only the Underlings stopped to talk to me. They were bumping along the surface, and so was I. They helped me to regain my breath.

I had been aiming too high. Receptionists, secretaries, porters, cleaners and orderlies were ignored as much as possible. Instead of reaching for the stars I should turn my eye to what was going on at ground level or below. I needed to get more literal. The power in any institution is in its basement. I visited the engine room to investigate the underpinnings. There was nobody around, but compressors still throbbed. Whoever was responsible for them was making what is supposed to happen happen, inconspicuously, and more effectively than the providers of patient care. I've never known the power system in a hospital to die (the talking shook its head at my bad joke).

At work I took the stairs rather than the lift. When I met the mainly Hispanic cleaners, and asked was there anything special that they wanted, they spoke up without fear or hesitation. 'I'd like a new bucket,' one said, 'the kind with a hole for the mop.' Another said, 'I'd like to learn to type so I can profit from my education. Not to throw in the cleaning job, but to supplement it. The pool is always short of typists. They fall in love and get married. I got married and fell out of love. And I have two children.'

Their sensible responses and lack of deference pleased me. I picked up a few Spanish phrases, such as 'una sonrisa no cuesta nada', a smile costs nothing, and it produced the desired effect. In the canteen a rat-like cockney in overalls told me, 'I do the drains.' I asked him if he was happy with the work. He said, 'It's satisfying in a way. But I would rather do chutes. Ever since I was a lad I loved climbing. Every other year after the leaves fall there is an accident. I apply to cover. But the boss isn't interested. Though what they really need is chap like me with a head for heights.'

The porter's lodge is the gateway between hell and heaven in a hospital. I took out my pipe with its St Peter, a small but perfectly formed man who had the power to decide entrances and exits. We smoked together. 'The job is my home. I was born to it, and have been here since. Everybody knows me, but nobody knows my name.' The lodge was a comfortable place to be, lived in and lived out. Jokes were exchanged, and gossip. I learned that his name was Christopher, and that the new Health Authority chairman, who was to prove no friend of mine, had been kicked out by his wife because he was having an affair with a trainee nurse. He was sleeping in his office. We both laughed as he was a bald, pompous man who drove a Bentley. A laugh costs nothing.

When Consultant Connie Domebaste was conducting some VIP visitors along a corridor where I was exchanging pleasantries with some Underlings, she paused and remarked snidely, 'Ah! Building up your constituency?' I pretended to be annoyed, but I was silently proud that the cleaners, orderlies, handymen and porters saw me as someone one could talk to. I had even got to know the names of their children.

My grass-roots strategy was not without effect. Small matters improved. The wearing of masks became compulsory for cleaners washing down the theatre with a new anti-HIV disinfectant whose fumes gave them migraines. A code of 'nice manners' was drawn up by the desk receptionists for patients and their relatives. They asked for the removal of the poster which had been issued all over the trust by the previous administration warning patients that if they didn't behave they would be thrown out by security. Phone etiquette was hotly debated. Should you stop talking to a patient at the desk to take a call, and keep them waiting, or risk offending someone on the line who might have a potential emergency? A more sympathetic switchboard was introduced. The sound of endlessly ringing phones was heard less. A friendlier atmosphere prevailed as the staff got on better with one another and, of course, with patients. There would be less angry shouting at the desk. Security men stopped playing at being bouncers, and were helpful rather than suspicious. Flowers began to appear in surprising places.

Union man Dick Cross took me to task for calling them Underlings. 'They are the Backbone.' He was interested in peer groups to improve their job satisfaction. Refreshments were laid on for lunchtime meetings. This was received with mixed feelings in higher places. A well-meaning Great and Good approached the Health Authorities to ask the Eminent Persons Group to propose a front-of-house policy. My advice was sought. I said that a policy existed ever since the caveman greeted potential enemies with a tree trunk to sit on. I talked to the local MP, Big Ben Newell, a friend of Dick Cross, and he spoke on morning radio about what to expect if you presented yourself as a patient in a hospital or clinic. 'The Have a Nice Day campaign is setting a gold standard for interpersonal relations. If it happened all over the country it would be tantamount to a revolution in medical manners. And it doesn't cost money. Una sonrisa no cuesta nada.'

I was wary when the Eminents started making nice noises in my direction. Dame Brenda met me accidentally-by-mistake outside my cubbyhole. 'So this is your piss-palace. Very engaging. Are you occupied?' She sat on my chair while I stood in the corner. 'Even Max is impressed by your grass-roots policy. You've come a long way despite… The group considers you a useful resource for testing the waters as things change. The outcome of the next general election is a foregone conclusion, and we're all New Broomers now. If you attended our meetings from time to time it would be of mutual benefit.'

Only one metaphor was significant. I was being ironed out but not ironised. But what she really wanted to know was if I was still talking to Mal Combes. I said, 'Not specially.' She smiled and lowered her voice, 'There is more purchase in talking to Stanley. He admires you in his fashion for sticking out your neck.' It gave me a chance to talk to Mal Combes. But his laugh was a mite forced. 'Watch it, Poet. Before you know it, you'll be an Eminent yourself.' I reassured him that I would always be his Trojan Horse. 'A theatrical one.' He laughed more easily. 'I will be the front end so we know where we're going. You'll be the backside so you can take the kicks.'

My head was spinning as I cycled along the Grand Union Canal. I was at a low ebb in my own mind, and yet it appeared I was riding high in the eyes of others. I stopped to talk to a fisherman who always gave me a wave. We talked about roach, perch, eels and minnows. That is, the fish he hadn't caught. 'I'm here for the beer,' he said, and offered me a can. Ungraciously I refused. 'Peanuts?' He offered me a bag and I took a fistful. Dame Brenda no longer saw me as a hummingbird, but I was still capable of flitting, and choosing the hand I ate out of. 'Keep going,' the fishless fisherman said as I pedalled off.

VII

RUNNING BACKWARDS
UP THE ESCALATOR

'Kindness is in our power. Fondness is not.'

—Samuel Johnson

STRATEGIC SYMPATHY

T HE STRATEGIC SLUMMING HADN'T PROVED JUST A distraction from whatever was playing havoc with my beautiful temperament. It was an upside-down fashion of observing things, and had led to self-suggested improvements, which the Underlings saw through themselves. All I did was pay attention, and it was reciprocated.

The Ground Forces were less amenable. No matter how hard I tried to be their friend I remained a necessary evil to them. Cassandra advised me to concentrate on renewing my visits to clinicians who were under surveillance due to complaints. 'Be nice to them. They need love.' She called it strategic sympathy. I thought of my father's wisdom: 'If we wish to show another that he errs we must notice from what side he views the matter, for on that side there is usually an element of truth.' I would be my father's son.

The dummy run, when I discussed the tea arrangements, was inauspicious, as the errants knew I had come to spy on them. Cassandra suggested that this time I should casually state the reason for my visit, and then talk of other things. 'Something personal, like where they live, or their mode of transport. Brief yourself in advance. Mrs Lucas and her clerks will know the low-down on family illnesses, fracases with colleagues, divorces, jewellery courses, gifted children, and difficulties at home. Underlying causes may be blurted out, and then you're on a roll. Larger issues can be tackled.'

Once again the staging of visits was theatrical. I rehearsed my performances with Cassandra. Because the script was unpredictable, on-the-spot improvisations were necessary. I made myself as small or big as the occasion called for – the personification of human sympathy ('There, there...'), or worse, empathy ('I know how you feel'). I calmed the unhappy with reassuring sentiments. My desire to avoid disciplinary hearings brought out in me the character actor with a hanky who, in the event of tears, turns away to allow the lead player the moment.

Anger could be mollified by conceding it was understandable. But righteousness had to be moderated. 'I'd probably do the same if I was in your shoes,' went with a shrug indicating it's an unjust world. 'But I would be wrong.' If they were political – left-leaning or ecologically inclined – I could sometimes find common ground by evoking Virchow. Damaged pride at someone jumping ahead of them on the career ladder could be soft-soaped by suggesting courses they might take, or offering sops like re-titling their job. Harry Huggins used special bonuses for malcontents. That everybody has a price is a fallacy. Most people have an *honour* price, which is best paid without money.

But sweeteners that appeared as a climbdown on the trust's part were anathema.

Practical suggestions meant more than sympathy. 'Take a holiday; I'll sort out your cover.' Or in extreme cases offering compassionate leave. And when they thanked me, I'd say, 'It's normal,' making a right seem like a favour. I was aiming at undying allegiance so they would bounce back, sooner rather than later, as paragons of the work ethic.

That it didn't always go according to plan is an understatement. I represented the 'violence without', and the 'violence within' was protecting itself from me. I'm not good at impasses. Impatience made me tear up the script, and thus lose the plot. The last resort was to offer suspension on full pay. Errants baulked at suspension. But when I emphasised that it was 'without prejudice' they left, unsure what it meant, or which side I was on. My hope was that this ambiguity would lead them to find another job. I waited a decent interval before sending the confirmatory letter on the off-chance.

'It's a dangerous game to play,' Cassandra said. 'Trust and sympathy do not always go together. In gaining the one, you may lose the other. Trust is what matters most in coming to an agreement that doesn't backfire.'

'So I have to be honest?'

'Yes, by hardening the heart, constructive dismissal can be avoided and progress made.'

'An honest bastard?'

'It can instil confidence by the back door. And, if you leave it open, sympathy can come back.'

'You're as bad as me.'

'Yes. Sometimes. But you're on a slippery slope with professional pride, and the associations in the background backing it. Counter-complaints are likely and then the floodgates will open. And do you want to be nearly drowned or nearly saved?'

STRATEGIC SINCERITY

I confined my clinic visits to delivering formal warnings, the first step towards a disciplinary. This challenged my principle of never giving up on my ideas ('Until it was too late,' said Mal Combes). The truth was I was miscast as Tartuffe. I was better at the gimlet eye than the deadpan. Joab agreed, 'You're too prickly.' But my ruling passion, embarrassment, made it easier to drop the curtain. Cassandra had pointed out that I was more interested in the reviews than the effect on my audience. I cared less about the outcome than my performance. And my performance was not convincing.

The experience had its bright side. Mal Combes's blank page on people to trust was underwritten by Conrad's: 'Falsehood lies deep in the necessities of existence, in secret fears and half-formed ambitions, in the secret confidences combined with an unspoken mistrust of ourselves' (*Under Western Eyes*). Becoming aware that nobody really trusted me was nearly enough to restore my faith in the dignity of man. I cherished the thought that, despite the Fall, mankind is no fall guy. The Seven Deadly Sins are balanced by the Seven Cardinal Virtues, and are topped by the eighth: 'Not being a fool.' Belief in the god of commonsense and humanity was possible. Something better could be hoped for, and not just for myself. Maybe Virchow was at the door on the night of the knocking.

I told Dr Jack that, 'despite Conrad and my devious inclinations, I trust myself, more or less. Now I must learn to trust others, in order that they trust me.' We agreed that it wouldn't be by empowering them, for power is fundamentally untrustworthy. But the sincerity would have to be strategic, as my job gave me power. 'Strategic sincerity,' he felt, 'could humanise you in the eyes of others, separating the title from the man. And, whether the sincerity is personal or pragmatic, nobody need know.'

But strategic sincerity would have its limits. Cassandra thought that it would frighten staff more than if I became a petty tyrant and laid all around me. 'Still, being straight with people will make you feel better. And for errants who fail to respond to your heightened honesty, there is always re-education and, that failing, dismissal is straightforward, and you will have achieved the opposite to what you intended.'

The strategy wouldn't work with crisis management as that is ultimately a matter of power. It would have to be ordinary, everyday. And nobody should be excluded from it. Still, that would be labour-intensive. I would have to multiply myself by several thousand to achieve a sincere rapport with all the staff. Rationing would be necessary. But merely picking and choosing the odd case wouldn't amount to a strategy. It would have to be trust-wide.

Strategic sympathy had taught me that an actor stands back from the emotions his audience is experiencing in order to concentrate on his technique. It's how they can live with their job. My compromise of a solution would be to generalise the personal, and distance myself, like Rostand's princesse lointaine, who cultivated *l'inertie,* leaving *l'enthousiasme* to others. I could then bask in a quiet life, feeling virtuous, having trusted people enough to let them get on with their responsibilities. It had worked with the Underlings.

My guiding principle would be Pascal's 'People only believe in that which they come upon by themselves'. But the ground would have to be prepared, and the appropriate seed made ready to plant so that the fruits thereof would be seen to be theirs, not mine. If taken to the ultimate I would be regarded as surplus to requirements. My Franciscan-like guru in the South Kensington training retreat would call it exit management. But I would stay on to reap my reward with a secure sinecure. I remembered that in my days of Ordinary Madness, Dr Hall McCall used to disappear off, saying, 'I leave you children to yourselves.' Jo Manders, and myself, worked to spite him. I was hoping my tactical withdrawal would have a similar response.

I thought I might try out strategic sincerity with the Eminents Group when Dame Brenda followed up her visit with a phone call. 'Stanley has proposed you come to our meetings on a regular basis. You would only be attending of course. Not that issues ever come to a vote. Only one proviso. Confidentiality. I think you know what I mean…' She did not need to finish the sentence.

I immediately spoke to Mal Combes, who said, 'Only a fool or you would bed down with that nest of vipers.' Then he gleefully remarked, 'Poet, as Dame Brenda would say, you're becoming a victim of your own success. But keep away from me. I'll let you know when it's time to call back the escalator.'

By accepting Stanley's invitation I was reacting to events that I couldn't fully understand. Whether it was a good or a bad thing, it would be interesting. I was strangely objective to myself and subjective to others. Maybe I was past caring about myself. If so, I was taking Socrates's 'second step to virtue', and Kierkegaard would have been proud of me. Bishop Berkeley might have given me the nod, saying something about my Christian concern for those I created (though surely I couldn't possibly have imagined the Eminent Persons Group all on my own?).

Philosophy has its consolations, and one of them is that nobody knows anything for certain. Hegel said accepting that was a philosophic duty. But perhaps my stand-off was just a good old-fashioned Kantian 'stand back' (wishful thinking thwarted, reason holds back from making a decision).

Meanwhile, every time I had to choose between taking an elevator or the stairs, Mal Combes's parting remark came to mind. Previously, I bounded up, three steps at a time. But now I waited for the escalator to descend, and allowed myself to be elevated. My fate was out of my legs.

THE STRUM

The night of the knocking could well have been Virchow bidding me farewell. In the cold light of dawn my stocktaking was sobering. I had pickaxed the surface with troubleshooting, disturbed the subsoil with peer review, patched up the financial footing so it wouldn't subside into cuts. However, I doubted my prefabrications would stand up to the aftershock of the seismic Sibyl. While the Established Order was attempting to reassert the ancient bedrock of the system, elsewhere creeping privatisation was gaining ground, even with the New Broom. Ambitious middle managers were reinventing themselves with crash courses in business studies. Newly formed companies were scrambling for consultancy work. Interest in the American health system included exchanges of visits by professionals. I could see on the horizon competitive tendering from multinationals for service takeovers. The talking shook its head sadly, 'How long, O Lord, how full of cant you are. A nation of shopkeepers is never going to go global.'

I took to visiting the Bright Young Specialists. It wasn't a matter of trust with them, but of mutual interests. They managed their training and development programme as a university outpost. I didn't discourage that as the trust held the budget, and Dean Slowey's patronage protected them (and me) from the Upper Echelons. We had lunches at the health-food cafe. They were all charmed by the owner's daughter Netta, who was full of life, but had sad eyes. Sometimes she sat in while we discussed Descartes and the fruits of the earth as the cure for all ills. Angus Cook brought her a bouquet of dandelions from Green Park, and asked her out. She said, 'You'll have to do better than that, my boyfriend brings me poems.'

After work the Bright Young Specialists were going to Ronnie Scott's Jazz Club and I joined them. Don Cherry was rumoured to be appearing. Angus took me aside and said, 'Watch your back. Everybody is waiting for something below the surface to bubble up. Before the government changes. The enemies of you-know-who see you as *his* weak link. But hold your ground. You're not without friends.'

Don Cherry hadn't turned up so Ronnie Scott was playing, and he was having problems with his teeth as usual. I was introduced to a jowly young man who recognised me quicker than I him. It was Murdock Gow, the youngest Eminent. The Bright Young Specialists were talking about the coming election. Angus said, 'The New Broom will want to scrap anything that has the

Sibyl's stamp on it, and our baby will be thrown out with the bathwater.' Murdock Gow shook his head. Angus mocked him, 'You are party to darkly mysterious forces…'

'Not least, Mal Combes,' murmured David Wills.

'Never heard of him,' joked Murdock Gow. 'But our friend here has.'

'Yes, he is a neighbour of mine.'

'We were all students of his, one time or other.'

'And everybody loves to hate him,' murmured David Wills.

'Except Nasty. She hates to love him,' gurgled Angus.

'I'm saying nothing,' I said.

Murdock Gow tapped me on the shoulder. 'I'll see you at the next Eminents meeting.'

'I don't know why I was asked.'

'The Lovecraft case rides again. They want you to deal with it this time.'

'But he's working in the private sector, and that's not regulated by Health Authorities.'

'Things are changing. Back as well as forwards.' But someone buttonholed Murdock before he could explain.

Ronnie Scott had stopped spitting into his sax. So I wandered off to see if I could spot Don Cherry. He was curled up in a corner playing his trumpet so softly only he could hear it.

As I returned I knew Angus was talking about me. 'Listen, he has the ear of Mal Combes, and Mal Combes has the ear of the Mandarins. He gets us bags of money so we can do what we want. You'd never think it but he's a political animal.'

'Brenda Tabby says he's a necessary evil,' laughed Murdock Gow.

'I like the necessary,' I said, 'but I am not sure of the existence of bags of money, or evil.'

'I thought Mal Combes is your neighbour,' murmured David Wills.

Angus mused, 'Throughout Mrs Sibyl's reign, Mal was a paid-up member of the New Brooms. Nobody knew about it, except Nasty, and perhaps Stanley. At college together in Leeds, they were young Broomers, old-style. Mal Combes is well-positioned to inherit the earth when the New Broom sweeps into power.'

The Don was, finally, persuaded to play for others. He had abandoned the trumpet, and cradled what could have been an Aeolian harp in his lap. 'Grazing Dreams,' he mumbled, 'music to sleep to.' He breathed on the strings and you could hear the hum (his or the harp's, who was to know the difference?).

FOGGING THE ISSUE

As far as the Eminents were concerned, it was clear I would have to content myself with strategic hypocrisy. Meanwhile, nobody in the trust noticed my strategic sincerity, except my faithful secretary Michelle. I was looking deeply into her eyes, and she said, 'I think you need glasses.' In the mirror I looked pathetic.

For the Ground Forces I was conspicuous by my absence, or as a fixed grin bypassed on the corridor, obviously going to some important meeting where I got them lots of money. In fact I wasn't up to much. Apart from the Eminents, there was not a lot happening. I was happy to let things drift ('As long as you do not know what is going on everything is alright'). A light wind behind me, and shelter, in case of a storm, was my aspiration. But the becalmed conditions were conducive to boredom, and so a phone call from Big Ben Newell was more than welcome. He wanted to know about the Bright Young Specialists.

His partner had benefited from their treatment, but he was surprised that she had been made a guinea pig for training. When I explained it was for the common good, he responded, 'This deserves publicity. Send me a press release.' I wrote one but it was dull with perspiration. I counted the words to make each sentence a word sonnet. This loosened up the doggedness that describing-work induces. But I was getting too literary for the *Evening Standard*. I called Joab and he introduced me to the Fog Readability Index. You choose words in common usage and vary their number of syllables according to what readership age you're targeting. I chose twelve-year-olds to ease the weary minds of commuters. My first attempt appeared with scarcely a word changed.

That is how I became my own public relations agent. I fed local papers tidbits of information about what was going on. Because the unsigned copy could not be traced back to me, I was reckless. References to scandals or urgencies that I made public were not uncommon during London Council election campaigns (I was Big Ben's pigeon). Editors liked my Fog style. It didn't need a journalist to revise. I suppose I was a pioneer of what is now called self-exploitation. Someone who does for free what makes money for others. Dick Cross wouldn't have been happy. The Virchow dimension didn't escape me. I was advancing my ideal by means that Machiavelli would have approved. But I had no control over the headlines. 'Rabies Is Rife in Brent' should have been 'scabies'. I was relieved no dogs were shot.

I was getting away with it in a small way. But, although my Trojan ponies for Virchow made easy reading for tired eyes, they had no larger impact. They left the general public unmoved. I had hoped that grass-roots lobbies would emerge. I put it down to language. Fog depended upon strict adherence to common parlance, and that was water off a duck's back. Brecht was right, I thought. 'If we don't change our vocabulary, it is underwear that never gets washed and, as poor hygiene is bad for the health, words end up as the dead bodies of things. Every word, new and old, ought to be given its chance. It's things that are dead.' My releases to the press began to be edited or even sent back as too fancy. However, by then I had exhausted anything that might cause a stir. So I stopped sending them before I was found out.

My addiction to verbal play took a new turn. I noticed a change in mores in the City. The young women in the eaves of the office buildings were no longer hookers, but secretaries out for a smoke. I coined a name for them, smookers, and, to bring the word into the language, I wrote a letter to the *Financial Times*, and also a piece for a social science journal, *ASSIGnation*. I'm still waiting for the dictionaries to catch up with me.

I spent my time rewording memorandums to be circulated, allowing myself the odd metaphor, and once a covert quotation from Montaigne ('There is merit in exchanging a bad situation for an uncertain one'). I had an urge welling up to use the word 'numinous'. A misprint for 'numerous' would be presumed. Readers rarely remarked on my caprices. No doubt they took it to be the latest jargon 'cascading down' from the Mandarins.

When the heating was on full in the wards despite a spring-time heatwave, my sly, 'You go into a hospital to be cured, not baked' went unremarked. But Max Madison spotted, 'Nothing continues to happen'. 'Did you really mean that? I think you're trying to be funny.' In the main nobody minded, if at all they noticed, my verbal play, except Ninette and Michelle who had to type and endlessly retype my Proustian amendments.

Joab calculated with Fog that the target reading age of my annual report to the Health Authorities was thirty-three, more than twice the recommended sixteen. But a Big Push with words was merely a diversion, which Pascal said was the sport of kings, and I was a republican. So I was relieved when the Mandarins sent a command from the government that all official documents were to be standardised according to a grid which made it easier for ministers to clear their red boxes. Each point would have a tick or a cross for the minister to circle. Even handwritten glosses on the page were becoming a thing of the past.

THE FASTEST RETURN CALL I EVER RECEIVED

In advance of the general election, money suddenly was found to renovate crumbling hospitals and clinics. Directors of works were recruited from the private sector for rosters of trusts. As they were regionally appointed, and represented new money, they commanded awe and respect. It was whispered that they were executives from the declining manufacturing industry, nobly opting for public duty in the interest of having a job. The first renovation by our director of works was his own office. I was tempted to add 'and Pomps' to his brass plate. Mother Hen Lucas and her chicks nicknamed him The Pasha. And it stuck.

The Pasha was busy negotiating outside contracts. He had rounds and rounds of meetings and lunches with business contacts. His status was enhanced by being hard to get hold of when staff complained of a broken compressor, or a leaking roof. You were made to feel a poor petitioner ('Affairs proceed at my convenience not your inconvenience'). Mrs Lucas wasn't the only one sorry that Jim Barrett of Estates had resigned ('to spend more time with my saxophone').

The Pasha judged your importance by the numbers waiting in the office to see you, the quality of your suits, and the make of your car. I met people mainly on the trot to avoid having to sit down; I wouldn't be seen dead in a suit (I have a codicil in my will); and worst of all, I rode a push bike. When I phoned him about something not done, and not done again, and eventually, after heroic persistence, got past his dead-bat secretary, he said, 'Put your complaint in writing.'

Before he could click off, I responded, 'But, of course. A *copy* will be on your desk tomorrow,' and hung up. The Pasha was quicker on his feet than me in realising from my unthinking use of the word 'copy' that I could be shopping him to some VIP at regional headquarters with a queue as long as Savile Row and a suit to match, who drove a Bentley, just like him. His return call was the quickest I ever got.

STANLEY O. KAY

Such successes by default are worth dwelling on. My response to The Pasha was unpremeditated, a verbal float. I had achieved much less with a lot more forethought. Not so for Stanley O. Kay, who had irons in so many fires, and Mal Combes, who was firing with so many irons. They always gave the impression that they were thinking of something else. In Stanley's case it could be the next shot at golf, and Mal Combes's the next kill. They were leaving you to do the thinking and, when you came up with an idea that suited them, you won their attention.

They also had in common crinkly grey hair and horn-rims, and a stature that was not imposing. Stanley O. Kay dressed the part of lord of the manor as to the manner born: tweed jacket, flannel trousers, and a dicky bow. Immaculate, as no doubt was his linen. Mal Combes's suits hung off him as though he'd got the buttoning wrong. Nasty said that he wasn't meant to wear clothes. 'He would have made a marvellous cannibal dancing around the pot.' Occasionally I saw him slinging a coat hanger with a suit draped in plastic on to the back seat of his car. And once when I asked him what was happening that weekend, he said, 'Nothing special.' I'd have loved to check if he was sporting matching socks and underwear. The Bright Young Specialists said women students from overseas had a weakness for him. I perished the thought as unworthy. He was no doubt dressing up for an away day with the New Broom.

Stanley O. Kay invited me to lunch to brief me on group meetings. He proposed his club, but I said I didn't have a tie, and suggested my rental health-food cafe. The staff were suitably attentive. Netta served. I asked her what was special about the dandelions today, other than the price? 'Angus picked them for me in Green Park, doctor. He calls them "dande-lines-of-poetry".' Stanley asked me what she meant. I said that it was a joke. He ventured, 'in that case wouldn't it be more modern to call you by your first name?'

Our tête-à-tête was like a mating dance. I played Gertie hard to get. He was vegetarian and offered to choose from the menu on my behalf. I refused politely, and ordered 'my usual'. Netta was perplexed. I hadn't eaten there before. Stanley said he'd have the same. She served us a mix of everything, including the dandelions. Stanley was solicitous that I try the carrot in beetroot juice, reassuring me that I could rely on his taste. I could see why Dame Brenda liked to say he was a safe pair of hands. I splashed beetroot over my shirt trying to imitate his forking. Dame Brenda knew about his hands. It was common knowledge that they once were an item until Max Madison came to rescue her on his high horse. I cherished the thought that the dark underbelly of the Eminents Group was throbbing with Grand Passions.

'Isn't he wonderful?' is the first thing that came to mind when you left Stanley O. Kay's company. Unlike Mal Combes, he didn't have a wife to pull him down a peg. 'Married to his work,' so said by everybody. Stanley was preserved in aspic. That was his camouflage, and giveaway. He didn't talk about matters pending. Wooing me with sweet nothings was his way of making clear that I must toe the line. Saying nothing was my way of acquiescing. When he asked me if I played golf, I felt recompensed. He was looking for a partner in a game I never played. I verbal floated, 'No, I haven't the plus fours for it.' His speech melody sounded disappointed. 'Funny, I always wear them.'

I accidentally-by-mistake bumped into Murdock Gow. I knew it was the Bright Boys' evening for Ronnie Scott's, and arrived before they finished work. He was also waiting and took me for a coffee, and without much prompting he spilled the beans on the two rivals. I hadn't known that Mal Combes had been an Eminent and then struck out on his own. When I said, 'Evidently there is no love lost between them,' he disagreed. 'They are the two sides of the same triangle, and the third is everybody else.'

'Everybody loves to hate Mal Combes, and hates to love Stanley.' (I was quoting Nasty.)

'Hate is ready money in this evil world. It is bankable. Stanley needs love and pays for it.'

'You mean he goes to…?'

'No. They come to him. And so do we all.'

Murdock Gow's account of the changing relations within the Established Order was beyond me. I had assumed Mal Combes's classification was hermetic. I hadn't reckoned with the 'osmosis of persons'. Apparently Stanley O. Kay and Mal Combes had friends in higher places, and therefore enemies. One step down, Dame Brenda and Max Madison had enemies in high places, and therefore friends too. The enemies were the same but not the friends. What Murdock Gow was telling me seemed obvious – a nod rather than a wink – until Angus arrived to take him to Ronnie's, and I was left alone to ponder who was who.

To clear my mind, I went to the Electric Cinema Club to see Erich von Stroheim's *Greed*. The film came out the same year that Stanley and Mal Combes were both born. The coincidence made me decide it was their story. Two prospectors in a gold rush where everyone is a law unto themselves, until it comes to the scales for the ore to be weighed, and greed is superseded. The true measure is pride. And it can only end badly. Having punctured one another's water bottles, it's a fight to the death in a desert storm while their gold dust is scattered to the winds…

But this time the butterfly of ambiguity did not alight. Not that the cinema had failed me. I had failed it. Instead of submitting to the film I had imposed my own cut, and it was specious. There was no real likelihood of Stanley O. Kay and Mal Combes cancelling one another out. They needed one another to roll on a plot that had no beginning or ending, only a middle. And

Murdock and me were stuck in it. The writing was on the wall but there was no difference to split.

On the Tube home I recovered myself sufficiently to see Stanley's game plain: uxoriously at home with himself, and his role as doyen of the Eminents, he saw the Established (Dis) Order as an opportunity to undermine Mal Combes's influence with the Mandarins by rejuvenating the membership. Murdock Gow was seen by them as the future. His work with the Bright Young Specialists and the peer review groups marked him out as a Consultant they could work with. Stanley had his eye on a few others, who had been Mal's students and were distancing themselves from him. I was co-opted to attend as I had a foot in the door at the department through Dean Slowey, not Mal Combes, who was looking increasingly isolated. Stanley's New Broom wouldn't be made from the bits and pieces of the old broom. He would graft on compliant new wood, partly by reducing Mal Combes's woodpile, until his handle on the Eminents was strong enough to maintain the broad sweep that would keep the procrastinations going. And, like Sherlock Holmes's study, the dust wouldn't be disturbed. But I could see Stanley in plus fours searching for his golf ball in the rough, and had my doubts that he would outmanoeuvre Mal Combes, who knew with Immanuel Kant that 'out of the crooked timber of humanity no straight thing can ever be made'.

Moreover, Stanley hadn't fully grasped that safety in numbers is passé. 'It's in everybody's interest' has no purchase if there is no such thing as society. Mrs Sibyl had announced its demise, and Little John, while mourning it, carried on as though it were true. And the New Broom would prove to be no different (indeed, closing down the National Institute of Social Work in

2003). If Lenin dreamed of a stateless society, Mrs Sibyl dreamed of a society-less state. Society was the enemy obstructing what politicians wanted to do. Dame Brenda loudly identified with this impatience. The people were the scourge of democracy, but they could be put in their place if you didn't offer them an alternative. Under Mrs Sibyl the culture of corporateness was strained, but now it was at breaking point. Stanley's dithering with power play by patronage was *démodé*.

I knew whose side I was on. The one I was least certain of. Mal Combes sometimes disowned me, and other times disappeared when I wanted him, but I felt more secure with his unpredictable support than with Stanley O. Kay's slippery blandishments. As a doer in a world that was not up to much, Mal Combes was principled by pragmatism. He revelled in Brecht's, 'We who try to do something, anything, we are the ones that all the crooked fingers are pointed at,' and disarmed his accusers by shaking hands with them, spitting on his palm before doing so.

THE EMINENTS' TRAP

At my first Eminents meeting I was made to wait while private business was discussed. I felt foolish having borrowed a tie for the occasion, and removed it before being called in. Murdock Gow gave me a good-luck wink. Dame Brenda was in the chair. I was given a corner seat and listened as they discussed the leaking of information on health service matters to the press. Had someone blown my cover? A code of conduct for whistle-blowers was discussed. It was decided to do nothing until a serious case arose. So far it had been trivial matters, scantily reported. It was agreed to advise reinforced confidentially for secretaries taking notes at meetings, or writing up minutes and reports.

The penultimate item on the agenda was on advice to the Health Authority. The ad hoc arrangement had not gone well. Group decisions needed time and Angela Khan's clerks kept ringing them up. Stanley O. Kay proposed taking turns as single advisors, starting with Murdock Gow.

The last item was me; or rather, Lovecraft. His resurfacing in Harley Street needed to be addressed. Dame Brenda said it ought to be reported to the Health Authority. But as the private sector was not in their jurisdiction, it would be necessary to revert to the complaints made when he was employed by the trust. Turning to me, she said, 'We will be advising them to revisit the case.'

'But I'm not the Health Authority adviser.'

'You were then.'

'The offences were not considered serious. Mainly cancelled operations. And putting a drop of oil of cloves on the noses of patients before examining them. His performance profile showed he was competent.'

'Whose profile?'

'Edna Gray's at the Reimbursement Board.'

'At the time her use of public information was not approved. It contributed to her early retirement.'

'She had cancer.'

'Nonetheless, it was illegal.'

'But it's legal now.'

'Not then. We will advise the Health Authority to take up the matter with the Medical Council, and *you*.'

'Does that mean I'll be called before the Medical Council?'

'By letting him go with a resignation you were putting private patients at risk. But if you hand over the dossier and cooperate it will probably save your skin.'

I looked hard at Stanley O. Kay. But he didn't flinch.

FALLING ON MY FEET FROM A HEIGHT

The New Broom, having promised to become a vacuum cleaner to suck up the mess left by Mrs Sibyl's legacy, gained power at last in 1997. Train disasters caused by crumbling infrastructure and 'die-ins' in hospitals made transport and health priorities. Money no object. The deregulated banks were flush from selling shares in the national debt (early days in what was a factor in the 2007–8 financial crash).

Mrs Sibyl had fallen on her sword, but she lived on in her successors. The New Broom talked up private/public partnerships, and other shareholder-driven schemes. Public services were 'failing' for lack of private investment. So money would be poured into them to make them more attractive to buyers. Tycoons and multinationals were rubbing their hands at the second coming of Mrs Sibyl in sheep's clothing. 'Would the increase in value be reflected in the price?' wasn't a question to pose. A joke circulating was that the famous 'flagship trust', Guy's Hospital, was asking for its tower block to be gold-plated.

There were changes in the mode of discourse. The Sibyl's warring metaphors, and Little John's pastoral rambles, gave way to the New Broom's populist analogies. They were a far cry from Plato's analogies of the cave and 'shared abstractions', or Proust's phantom analogies 'that let us escape from the present'. A sampler might read something like, 'The middle-of-the-road vehicle of efficiency, effectiveness, honest endeavour, is road-worthy. So we will get to where we want to be by kick-starting the ground rules set by our patriotic duty. The bottom line is it will save money which can be used to top up the quality of life.'

But all analogies are mirages. The simulacrum can't substitute for the real thing any more than the part can equate with the whole. What falls into place is the illusion, in this case of progress. The rhetorical scaffolding holds up rickety half-truths. The big idea is the little idea. Virchow seemed as remotely unlikely as Lenin's promise of a stateless society.

Everybody was working on the hop, myself included. And now that the 'crooked finger' was being pointed at me, it was time to point it at myself. I came to change things, but things had changed me. If I cooperated I would keep my job. All that would be expected of me was that I functioned. My edge would gradually be reduced to a tailor's pin in the remodelled emperor's new clothes of the Established Order.

I wasn't even dancing with the devil. Rings were being run around me. The Eminents may have been fighting amongst themselves, but I united them in a small way. Being a pawn in Mal Combes's chess game wasn't flattering, but it was a humiliation worth the risk. But with Stanley's golf, not knowing his game, my playing a puffball in the rough might lead to an existential embarrassment or the re-enactment of the end of *Pierrot le Fou*. I suppressed the urge to counter them by playing games of my own in order to save myself further embarrassment. My mother's son, I threw myself back into hyperactive management, interfering with day-to-day matters with more sincerity than sympathy.

I was the lowest common denominator of a petty official. I who once had world historical ideas.

The next meeting of the Eminents was an anodyne affair. All was sweetness and light. Lovecraft wasn't mentioned, until 'Any Other Business', and then merely to say it would be on the agenda next time. I knew what was expected of me. When the date of the next meeting was agreed I gave my apologies: 'I will be on holiday,' I lied. Dame Brenda remarked that it was probably not the best of times to be sight-unseen. I explained that it was a tactical ploy to put my staff on their mettle. I was hoping they'd rise to my absence. Dame Brenda gibed, 'Whose idea was it?' 'My shrink's,' I replied (and, indeed, it was Jack's). She laughed rather too loudly. 'Mal Combes, the mind doctor. You've been brainwashed. But don't overestimate your low achievers.' Stanley intervened, 'We'll put Lovecraft on the agenda when you come back.'

After the meeting he took me aside and said that they had been looking at the quality standards produced by peer review. They left something to be desired and the group would be fine-tuning them for the Medical and Dental councils. I was left with the distinct feeling that I was being edged out. Although I had already made myself surplus to requirements with Dean Slowey's specialists. But the unspoken, as he surprised me by shaking my hand, was Lovecraft.

ON THE ALTAR OF LOVECRAFT

I was idling. That does not mean I wasn't doing my job. I was doing it without thinking beyond the detail in hand. The functionary was functioning. Ever-present in the workplace, I couldn't be faulted for timekeeping. My dumb-focus had narrowed to the point of application. I cleared my in tray and waited for the next post.

As the Ground Forces got used to my hands-on management the necessary superseded the evil. Even though I was a fusspot, I could be depended upon to fight their corner with the Powers That Be. However, should I become a plaything of the Eminents that could lead to a conflict of interest. And I didn't want to live with contradictions again. The night of the knocking was a watershed. I detailed the conflicting pressures to Dr Jack, and he recommended a career break: 'Why not attach yourself to a peace-keeping mission in Africa? There is a sore need for aid workers there.' Still, larger ideas were out of the question. I had to think small to keep sane. But when he saw my dead bat, Dr Jack added, 'You Irish are good at keeping the peace, *except* in Ireland.' He had crossed the barrier between thinking and saying, which for an Englishman is an expression of friendship. I felt the better for it.

The knocking didn't return, but I slept less and less, getting out of bed to scribble little notes to myself to remind myself of things or people to be done, squared, squashed or whatever. The self-writing had been replaced by the devil of detail. Pounding the floorboards at all hours, it was dawn before I got uninterrupted sleep. Once I dreamed of Mal Combes's remark about calling back the escalator. I was at the bottom of the stairs with all the world returning backwards to trample me. As though by telepathy, I was woken by a call from Mal Combes: 'Poet, you may not realise it, but you've done me a good turn. You're setting up the Eminents to fail, to coin a phrase. They think you are the whipping boy, the Turk's Head. But be assured it isn't your head that's going to roll. Stanley had taken you to his heartless bosom, but you have knocked him off balance, and Dame Brenda and Max Madison have pulled the carpet from under him by raising the stakes with the Lovecraft case. Find a pretext for seeking his advice, and phone me.'

I ignored my Abraham. If I was to be sacrificed on the altar of Lovecraft, it would not be as a lamb. I took the dossier to Angela Khan, and she said it would be old hat soon. The odd private sector scandal was making the news in the court reports as usual – a dentist accused of assaulting a patient under a general anaesthetic, a gynaecologist who misdiagnosed a false pregnancy. These were the tip of the iceberg, Angela said. 'The Medical Council are under pressure to accept that private cases within Health Authority boundaries are their responsibility. It was only a matter of time.' She had convened a meeting with the council using Lovecraft as a test case. 'You will be invited to attend without prejudice.' 'What does "without prejudice" mean?' I asked anxiously. 'Bring an Eminent with you if you can. It will be an eye-opener.'

As I left I asked her how the Eminent advice went. 'It is a nightmare. Everything takes so long, and they have such loud voices.' Then I mentioned Murdock Gow. I said he would be quicker than me, and he talked sense. And I was hoping, since I couldn't be my own Trojan Horse, he would be mine. She said, 'Don't count on it.'

PART THREE

VIII

TIME TO REMEDITATE
ON LIFE AND LOVE

*'The outside world is too small, too clear-cut, too truthful,
to contain everything a person has room for inside.'*

—Kafka

LEAVE WELL ALONE

OVERDRIVE MEANT OVEREXPOSURE. BLAKE'S 'DEAR
Mr--- did it ever strike you/ the more I see of you, the
less I like you' could have been me. My reputation as a benign
presence had not been enhanced by a disciplinary case that
came back to haunt me from my troubleshooting days. Dr Lisa
Lemming had resigned when the writing was on the wall, and
was now claiming constructive dismissal. She was a popular
member of staff (her Christmas parties were said to be the event
of the year). Her offence was prescribing a drug for epilepsy
to a woman with postnatal depression. As legal costs would
be prohibitive, I was being encouraged to settle out of court.
This I was resisting. I feared the floodgates would open from
the days when ridding or redeploying ineffectual employees

was my main strategy. I wanted to be nearly drowned, not nearly saved.

I should have followed Kierkegaard's advice to the King of Denmark when his popularity was at a low ebb: 'Get sick.' But that was before Koch postulated the germ theory of disease. Now most common ailments are identifiable. If I fell sick without a specific diagnosis it would be considered psychosomatic, and that would be seen as a weakness. I didn't have confidence enough in my charges to submit myself to possible scorn. I thought, though, an accident might do the trick. People liked to warn me of the risks of cycling in central London, and they would be pleased to be proved right. I perished the thought. However, I could fake one as I did in my days in Mach's army. But dislocating my double-jointed elbow might do more harm than good. The old joint wouldn't leap out of its socket so readily as in my careless youth.

I cancelled for the second time the last of the disciplinary hearings pending. It was one in which I suspected there were extenuating circumstances. Cases that were not cut and dried invariably plunged me into an abyss of a deeper dye than blatant offences (theft, violence, criminal negligence). I couldn't face the black-hat moment when, one way or another, the judgement would be thrown back in my face. In this case I was waiting for the errant's marriage to break up. 'Mrs Lucas said it could lead to a job change too,' I told Cassandra, who listened to me with patience, and suggested I take a holiday, pointing out incidentally that I'd lose three years of untaken leave if I didn't.

OLD FRIENDS

I stayed in London undercover (keeping off my beaten tracks). I wanted to renew contact with friends I had been neglecting. I resumed my Sunday evenings with Ian Russell, ranting on about my job. But as it made him nod off, and I found myself talking to myself, I took more interest in his life. Ian had recently divorced his wife, but not his two children, and the three lived next door to his apartment. It was possible to be friends. There's hope for the god of common sense and humanity, I thought. I asked after Madge Herron. And he said that she had disappeared. 'Maybe she has become the bag woman she always pretended to be.'

I had mislaid the addresses of people I knew in my days of Ordinary Madness. The exception was McFee, my ex-landlord philosopher (see: *Light Years*). I knew it off by heart. I learned that his dizzy first wife Eliza had run away with a Russian Orthodox priest, but he had remarried. Fay was easy going, and they, despite scant money, and too many children, exuded a happy complicity.

McFee was still the eternal student, speaking in quotations. 'Life is flipping the pages of a book backwards. As quickly as you turn a few pages, like an old person with their memories, you can meet yourself in the flight from the present.' His grand statements were like Pascal's sneezes, and I made a wish. In no time it came true, and we were back twenty years 'absorbing all the functions of the soul'. I was twenty-six again and bog ignorant, though I didn't know it.

'"You may not have visible means of support," I said, "but you have invisible ones."'

'I forgot, you studied under the master.'

'Yes, I owe Søren Kierkegaard to you, and probably some back rent as well.'

'That's forgotten too.'

'He saved me from myself.'

'And from getting married.'

'What has he done for you?'

'He taught me to live forwards and think backwards. And while my life will have a conclusion, there will be no end to my thinking.'

'Or your doctoral thesis,' teased Fay.

'My philosophy is still in the process of clarification. Kierkegaard said that, "Man cannot stand outside the movement of life and understand it." And so no philosophic system can ever be complete. My thesis remains an unfinished work. I study to no end except to study things which cannot be understood.'

'So we bask in ignorance?' I intruded.

'Far from it. "We know what we don't understand." Socrates.'

'In the dark then.'

'Yes, but we know where the light switch is. According to Kierkegaard there is a different kind of understanding other than thinking backwards. Understanding that comes with the movement of life which obliges us to qualify our thoughts and make decisions.'

'In other words we seize the moment and get something done. That's Hegel.'

'Who Kierkegaard called von Jumping Jack. But no. We seize the moment and do nothing.'

Fay smiled over the woolly pullover she was knitting.

'And what do you do for a living, my young friend?'

I spoke about Virchow and my dream of a Nietzschean 'reversal'.

'What the object thinks of its user, the landscape thinks of the sightseer, the horse thinks of its rider,' said McFee.

'What the body thinks of the mind. It's Descartes's politics by other means. The assumption of health as the supreme power ruling mankind.'

'It sounds like medical fascism to me.'

'No. It's common sense.'

'Putting Descartes before the horse of instruction won't get you anywhere when faced by the PIG8O of Wrath.'

'Ah! Your Post-Industrial Global Oligarchy. Where politics and big business meet to trap workers and peasants worldwide into being consumer slaves in order to be satisfied with more of less.'

'I blame television,' said Fay. 'The year it came to Italy, I was backpacking by train from Sicily to the mainland across the Strait of Messina, and saw the peasants throw away the rye bread and cheese and dig into cellophane wrapped cookies, and their wine turned into Coca-Cola.'

'Coca-Cola is the premier product of PIG8O,' said McFee. 'It started out a cocaine stimulant and ended up a fizzy sugar drink. People don't know what's good for them, and health is the last thing they think about. You're wasting your time.'

'But nothing comes from doing nothing,' I said weakly.

'It's done me no harm.'

'If I had done nothing too,' said Fay, 'we would not be together.'

'Do you know our song is, "And you'll know at a glance by the two pair of pants".'

'Know what?'

'"When my love comes along". It's from *Guys and Dolls*. When the Russian Church stopped having their masses in the parlour room, I rented it out to the local light-opera group, and that's how I met Fay.'

'What do the two pair of pants signify?'

'Someone boring with a change of pants for a steady job.'

'I got the wrong man,' said Fay. 'Or got the man wrong. He's not a doer.'

'"Doing, a filthy pleasure is, and short."'

'Ben Jonson,' I said. 'But thanks for giving me a poetical basis for what I wanted to forget.'

'What?'

'Getting things done.'

'Keep forgetting.'

As I left Fay gave me a hug.

On the stairs I was met by a stampede of children. The next generation of McFees wore school caps and uniforms.

I had kept up with Joab by phone for intellectual emergencies. All I knew of his personal life was that he said he was suffering a worsening choice in women. Hard to believe, after Andrea, the hoyden from Croyden, who wore black body stockings and was a late-onset Madonna fan. But his string of love had no end. He wanted me to meet Shusha. I knew what that signified. Ridding himself of another mistake by downgrading her to a friend's friend. Joab this time was more direct: 'I'd like her to think she's dumping me, it's less messy. I'll discuss a movie on in the Electric which I know she won't have seen. Neither will you, and you'll ask her to come with you.' Remembering Andrea's drunk and disorderly performance, I revolted, 'I've nothing against Truffaut's *Jules et Jim* except Jeanne Moreau's singing. But, Joab, what do you take me for? A dump truck for your throw-outs?'

I went to see Dr Jack, instead. He was just back from Bosnia where he was counselling widows and orphans and didn't want to talk about it. I told him I had been thinking about the rice-rat study into ageing, and it had given me second thoughts about Virchow. 'If investment in health was boundless, technical advances eventually would prolong life indefinitely. The world would become populated by oldies sustained by medicine, with an ever-diminishing capacity to procreate. And so mankind hoisted on Virchow's petard would degenerate into Swift's Struldbrugs, a debilitated species awaiting its extinction...'

Dr Jack demurred, 'Virchow, as a humanist, would anticipate that by maintaining a troupe of vestal virgins, and a sperm bank.'

'I'm not sure the earth could sustain a population explosion of old people even if it had the young to work it.'

'The power of medicine could never eliminate one side effect of living: normal wear and tear. Virchow would see to a balance between birth control and natural deaths.'

'I hope you're right. The thought of mankind as a race of geriatric fitness freaks fighting the good fight against the dying of the light is almost as horrible as the idea of living forever. That is more frightening than the fear of death.'

'Say that to the people in a war zone.'

I confided to him that the talking in my head had ceased since I had taken a break.

'That means ambiguity is absent without leave, and you're beginning to live. Profit from it.'

Congol O'Curry of the One Ball Gang had recently run away from his large family with an American post-graduate student, and settled in Putney. Holly answered the phone, and I could catch them discussing whether to invite me down or not. I had been mistaken for my brother, Michael, now unbelievably a priest. I didn't disenchant him, saying that I was on my way to Rome to research Little Nellie of Holy God in the Vatican archives. His 'Say hallo to the Pope' was not cordial.

I hadn't been in touch with Tim and Jill Labrinth since my troubleshooting days, but they were glad to see me. 'You haven't aged a day,' they said in unison. Liars, I thought, beloved liars. In the bathroom mirror I looked like van Geloven, the serial killer. At the fairground in Graball Bay I once tried to kiss Jill. She was now a far cry from the timid girl who said, with tears in her eyes as she pushed me away, 'Sorry, I'm already spoken for.' Later that summer, observing the mackerel boats from above the Blue Pool in Myrtleville, I caught sight of Jill and Tim on the rocks below, hand in hand, and bit my lip.

Jill was now a Euro MP for the Greens with a power suit and trenchant views to match. I was tempted to say there was nothing wrong with lead in petrol. But I could see that Tim was just about holding his own with her, nodding agreement when she spoke. Instead I talked about Descartes's 'fire, water, air, sky, stars' and, as she looked bored, diversified to his herbal remedies ('Savouring the fruits of the earth, and all its comforts, to preserve our health').

She was on the board of the homoeopathy hospital. I said nothing about being party to a lobby who wanted to turn the listed building into a medical museum. The staff would be rehoused in the university hospital where their treatments could be scientifically tested. Needless to say, nothing happened as they were protected by royal patronage. I merely remarked, 'The

homoeopathists sport the best beards and tweeds in England.'
She was willing to be amused, as it was true.

I was surprised to learn that Tim didn't have a job commensurate with his youthful brilliance. He was still teaching English
in a technical college in Hatfield. 'I do some editing of facsimiles
in the British Museum, and I coach children at tennis.' Then
I remembered his famous essay on Coleridge's poem, 'Work
without Hope' and Leibniz's *optimisme*. Tim concluded that the
poet's 'work without hope' being 'honey in a sieve' meant you
ended up in a dead-end job, and with Leibniz's 'hope without
an object' you got stuck in the mud. I was sure his 'hopes' had
attained their 'object'.

None of the friends that I visited appeared to have considered
themselves neglected. It was as though I had never been away.
This ought to have pleased me. Forever present. But I died a
little, wondering why they thought so little of me that they left
three years go by without contacting me. As I took my leave
of the Labrinths, feeling it was neither here nor there to them
whether they saw me again, Tim lingered at the door and said
thoughtfully, 'It's been too long, my old friend.'

'So you missed me?' I said bluntly, and he echoed my words,
but more softly.

'Until the next time,' he sighed.

My social skills had been impaired by a closet existence. I
was capable of holding two emotions simultaneously – my
resentment, and Tim's regret – and allowing them to cancel one
another out. I should have embraced him. Instead I promised to
come back soon, knowing I wouldn't. I was convinced that with
my friends I was what Hegel called 'a finite concern, welcome
but not essential'. They wouldn't mind if I left it forever, having

full lives of their own with children, careers, gardens, dogs, and the stuff of domestic contentment. Reality had taken over from the ideal.

TRANSPORT

As I rode off on my bike I felt anger against myself. No less than me, my friends experienced ordinary unhappiness. More so, as they had the courage to engage with family life. There is never enough love to go around and, spread too thin, it dissipates into separations and even divorces, and the apparently settled ends up in rancorous settlements. Then I thought of McFee. When the love of his life ran away with a patriarch, he was philosophical, and found a chorus girl with whom he could live an idea. In their case happiness is not an amateur concept. It's a release from guilt that puts pleasure before pain. The common good is to be found in the mixed pleasures of the mind and bringing up children. It is utilitarian rather than utopian, and provides shyly a Benthamite analogy for my murky career that cheers me up.

How my friends got around the town summed up how they had changed. Tim had a car that ran on alcohol, an eco-experiment. McFee sometimes accompanied Fay with her pram. Joab Comfort's Ford Escort, the one that Andrea had wrecked, had been replaced by an identical model. Congol and Holly had matching super-scooters, and no doubt he was ashamed to learn how they work. Ian Russell preferred to walk, or jog. He was looking after himself. Me? A functional hybrid had replaced the musical Mayday Raleigh, stolen in my days of Ordinary Madness. A loss I have never recovered from. Every time I threw my leg over the bar to land on the pedal cleat I missed the harmonious relationship my body had with that old wife of a push bike (a bit heavy on the steel but, because of the low-slung saddle, the handlebars were an embrace).

My Mayday Raleigh was made for the terrain. The high-impact fibre body of the hybrid, half-racer, half-mountain bike, was lighter, but a less comfortable ride on the towpaths of the Grand Union Canal, or when kerb-hugging on London streets. If you deviated into the gutter you got punctures. The Mayday defied the reckless couriers who zigzagged through the furious traffic with no respect for anyone's safety. I kept to the slipstream, taking my chances. But I hadn't the same freedom of the road with the hybrid. City drivers made me feel a threatened species and a hated one. Once a big dog leant out the window of a car and bit me.

LONDON IRISH LOSE

I haunted places where I would bump into people from my youth. For example, the Grapes of Wrath, the pub for Irish graduates. In the late 1990s it was still packed with doctors and dentists and their hangers-on from the lower reaches of the humanities (commerce and pass arts). The drink was still going strong. I talked to those still recognisable and, not knowing what to say, I asked them their children's names. The most common were indeed Rory and Maeve, the last king and queen of Ireland. Exchanging names of children and/or dogs is the lowest form of intimacy, but it enhances friendly feelings between strangers. Renewing contact with my coevals saddened me. They didn't for the most part look healthy or happy. But they made an effort to be convivial, slapping backs and sharing jokes. Old age was creeping up on us, and we were in the anteroom to the unknown.

Those with degrees in the professions tended to marry one another. This happened when they first came to London. It wasn't just falling back on what they knew. It made good yuppie sense. In the Grapes of Wrath the wives were conspicuous by their absence. I wondered how many of such couples were 'staying together for the sake of the children'. I perished this beady thought, and asked after their wives whom I'd often known as girls. 'Elaine couldn't come tonight. She has her knitter-natter group,' 'Breda has turned into her mother,' and so on. The banter was forced. I said to a financial journalist, who from childhood was Little Larry to me, 'I don't think us old friends like one another any more.' He told me everybody was a bit down as London Irish lost. I asked myself, 'What do we know about people?' (Marlene Dietrich at the end of Orson Welles's *Touch of Evil*). But it wasn't a bad rugby result that made me leave early. I saw myself in the Guinness mirror and someone I half-recognised behind me, his beard in his beer. We could have been ageing twins. I had turned into Turlough McGee, the dodgy insurance man.

At the Irish Club I met the well-heeled businessmen who would have liked to go to college, and the engineers. Their lackeys were rather unexpectedly artists and writers, poets in particular. It wasn't just for the drinks. Their wives were often vultures for Irish culture. The walls of the restaurant were crowded with pictures, and they were bought, particularly when the artist was sitting at the table. Yeats's Rhymers Club lingered on. Poets were paid, and performed under the patronage of George Buchanan, an old charmer once famous for his poetry and plays. The audience was exclusively ladies in hats.

But I wasn't looking for the literary scene. In my youth I had mingled enough amongst the egos. I needed human contact and warmth. I was recognised by a friend of Tim, a Celtic scholar called Thomas O'Kane. He now worked in advertising. He introduced me to his Welsh wife, Rowana, a designer, who dead-eyed me. She was engaged in flirting with a florid giant called Rory, who on hearing my name descended on me with an all-embracing thump. His pint of Murphy's frothed with emotion, as he recalled college and the One Ball Gang ('now all famous'). He had been on their fringe. But his poems had been scorned for resembling Keats. His secret influence though was Rilke. He had a German dictionary and translated word for word some of the less known sonnets without acknowledgement. When he was invited to read with us at the Maple Leaf tea room, I was fooled by the Rilke but not my friend, Hugh J. Murphy (who had moved on from his landlady to a German bluestocking): 'Shame on you. And you're a policeman's son?' But Hugh J. and myself, as the mainstays of the Lee Road Anarchist Society, were not ideologically disapproving.

Now I recalled Rory plain. A broth of a boy who studied in the valley bar. The pint glasses piled up on the table before him. When asked what he was reading, he would say the law. I remembered his father, a point policeman who kept the traffic flowing at the junction between the quays and Patrick Street.

'The last of the great moustaches,' I said.

'Yes. I learned all I needed to know about the law from him,' Rory said, almost seriously. Tom O'Kane later told me that he was the richest Irishman in London.

'What in?'

'Antiques at the moment, but it wasn't always so.' I didn't know what to make of that, and as I made my manners and left I heard someone say, 'Who was that?'

I continued collecting children's names in the Irish University Club, essentially an out-of-hours drinking establishment for my fellow countrymen. Curiously, I found that while the boys, by and large, retained the expected traditional ones like Patrick, Conor and Kevin, there was a preponderance of Greek goddesses amongst the girls. Apart from a loose change of Pennys, and Danaës, my list included a Clio, Diana, Flora, Jocasta, not to mention a Juno. I was talking about this to the parents when an eavesdropper shouted, 'Ah! The boys are all saints and the girls sinners.' It was Rory, and he began to recount the iniquities of the classical divas, until someone stopped him. 'There are ladies present.' I felt at home with the laughter, but wondered should I ask Hervě Thuau, my anthropologist friend, to investigate this phenomenon? I perished the thought. He would want to open the Pandora's box of mixed marriages and divorces, and an Irish Catholic myth about families would be compromised. The laughter was sufficient.

I met Noel O'Connell, the secretary of the Irish Texts Society, a financial adviser of evident culture. I mentioned I had been a member since 1916. He asked for my name. 'Ah, yes, the hereditary subscriber. Your address has been the subject of some consternation. The latest volume came back, recipient unknown.' My patrimony was in good hands. Solid green scholarly editions of the Gaelic poets and sages had blocked my letter box every third year. Alas, as my Irish declined from lack of use, the solid green volumes with gold leaf titles remained decorative rather than read.

Sated with Irish affability, barbed or genuine, I dropped in on the Poetry Society in Earls Court, where Netta was said to be moonlighting at the bar making health-food cocktails. I introduced myself to the loners on high stools as a friend of Ian Russell. As an *entrée* that worked. Everybody knew him. And wanted me to know them and their books which were on display on a table behind me. I explained I was doing a survey of children's names. The bar became animated. I wrote down Daphne, Phoebe, Phyllis, and a smattering of colour-coded names like Amber, Jade and one Pinkie. I asked after Netta, and was told she was now in PR with Lord Sachs of Money. I didn't believe it. My last conversation with her was about a return to barter, everybody foraging the earth for natural products. I said goodbye to the poets. Their world had no loose threads for me. I'd have to stitch myself into the rather fragile tapestry of lives dedicated to being neglected and underappreciated, and at the same time glorying in it. I thought of Madge, and revisited her Tufnell Park bedsit. But the house was being demolished to make way for gentrification. A neighbour said Madge was living rough. She was last seen on the Victoria Embankment. Apparently she was not unhappy. 'That's what she always wanted to do.'

I made a point of dropping into the health-food cafe/shop and was told Netta was engaged to Angus Cook. So the dandelines-of-poetry had worked.

IX

FIRING ON ALL CYLINDERS

'Nothing happens by chance.'

—*Zadig ou la Destinée*, Voltaire

HUMAN CONSIDERATIONS

I PHONED INTO WORK A WEEK BEFORE I WAS EXPECTED
back. Nobody had missed me, or so Michelle said. At first I felt
pleased. My tactical withdrawal had worked, or so it seemed. But
my satisfaction was tinged with a soupçon of resentment. Not
being missed is to be 'a finite concern, welcome but not essential' (*pace* Hegel). This double thinking alerted me to a possible
premature return. I had my reasons. Most particularly I needed
to do something, anything.

Michelle had sorted my mail for Mrs Lucas and her clerks
to deal with. Nothing was pressing, except Mrs Manders. Jo
wanted to talk to me about an article I had revised for her
ages ago, 'Dentures in the Trees'. Now retired, the mother
was back living with her. Haddie had been thrown out of
Last's Resting Home. Her dementia had become dangerous
to others.

240

I cycled across the Heath to visit them. A pity it wasn't our furious piece about madness and the focal-infection scandal, I thought. In the 1920s Henry Aloysius Cotton, an American neurosurgeon, removed the large bowel from numerous patients in mental institutions, having decided it was the focus of insanity. Stanley O. Kay was writing a book about the history of medicine. A copy of *It's a Mad, Mad World* would give me a pretext to talk to him. I wanted to ask him to accompany me when I spoke to the Health Authority about Lovecraft. I needn't have bothered. He had already invited himself.

The Manders lived in a doll's house in Hampstead Garden Suburb, or rather a cottage built on an *Alice's Adventures in Wonderland* scale. Jo greeted me brusquely, 'Where have you been?' and before I could answer told me about the squirrels in the attic. She had put down rat poison and you could hear them drop dead, she said. Haddie, in the corner by the stove, smiled docilely, and apart from dribbling into her bib, didn't look like the third oldest woman in England. Jo Manders read my mind. 'She has achieved a permanent vegetative state, and when I want to go on a cruise I put her in the deep freeze.' Haddie cackled. I had no doubt she understood every word.

In the corner there was a fish tank. A long black eel-like creature flicked its tail at me. It was a piranha. Jo said, 'It keeps Haddie happy. They eyeball one another for hours on end.' A perforated roof had been installed to prevent her dipping her finger in. I asked, 'What do you feed it?' Jo muttered, 'Anything that lives.' 'Mice?' I hazarded. 'Rats more likely.' And she changed the subject to 'Dentures in the Trees'. She wanted to have it published, and thought it might be suitable for *Reader's Digest*. After several further revisions – Jo didn't see the point in punctuation – it was to appear in *The Probe* as part of a planned series which would include false teeth for sheep and tooth implants for wind-instrument players (in memory of Ronnie Scott). We parted amiably. Haddie threw me a last lethal kiss.

I wasn't to enjoy such Ordinary Madness again. All the functions of my soul were being absorbed, not with a sneeze but with the hiccups. The deep-dye disciplinary case that had been left to drift in the hope that it would just go away, hadn't. Divorce didn't conquer all. A new life elsewhere was not going to be. Worse, the Lisa Lemming complaint for constructive dismissal was in the hands of the solicitors. Dr Agata Brun, her friend and colleague, was bad-mouthing me wherever she could. Max Madison, who had qualified with her father, rang me up, and said it would end badly for me. But I couldn't risk a settlement. Cases that had been found alternative jobs would get the whiff of compensation. Cassandra sighed. 'So you'll end up in the tribunal. Your enemies will be pleased.'

'Not if someone could persuade the patient prescribed an epilepsy drug for postnatal depression to take out a case.'

'Against who?'

AMEN

Stanley O. Kay turned up to my meeting with the Health Authority at the last minute. MacCrone, the mystery Mandarin, just happened to be there. There was no one from the Medical Council, which augured well, I thought. Angela Khan said she would speak for them. 'The most recent complaints against Lovecraft – about fees – have been withdrawn.'

'He must have paid them off,' said MacCrone.

'But the original accusations still stand. Edna Gray's findings in favour of his performance can be challenged. At the time her index had not been confirmed by independent research, although it has been since. Stanley will explain.'

'The human factor that makes for the best and worst of care can't be quantified. Numbers only show up numbers. But adjudging quality without standard criteria is unprofessional. The distinction between *mistreatment* (nobody is perfect) and *maltreatment* (criminal neglect) must be clear. Only in extreme cases like war is there one. Fortunately we have no need for body bags...'

'As of yet,' said MacCrone.

'Quality guidelines already exist on paper through Slowey's audit group. But since the Dean retired, we are reworking them. The Delphi Method will be deployed in a double-blind questionnaire to reach as close to a consensus as possible. We will be using international experts already engaged by medical insurance companies. Litigation has not yet become anything like it is in America, but it's only a matter of time. Dame Brenda knows that, and she sits on the board of MedSure.'

'So the Eminents will be the oracle of quality?' said MacCrone.

'No. Everybody from the Medical Council to the lowliest clinician will be singing from the same hymn sheet.'

'Hallelujah,' said MacCrone.

Angela Khan addressed me. 'Since you dealt with the case you will be called on to give evidence.'

'But everybody has seen my dossier.'

'A verbal hearing will be necessary. You will be questioned on a possible error of judgement. Though the subsequent tests on the index have showed it is reliable, with a ninety-five per cent probability of predicting an errant.'

'I've nothing to add, except it appears I was wrong to be right. But I will cooperate, of course.'

Afterwards Stanley shook my hand, and murmured, 'Well done.'

'Amen,' said MacCrone.

I walked through the night, an active form of insomnia. It is possible not to think. And I faced the dawn in an all-night cafe with vagrants and vice workers. I felt I was a bit of both. Nobody spoke. It was a communion of sinners, I thought. I smiled passively at the trickle of night workers having a fry-up before bed. They nodded and turned away.

If embarrassment was the outward expression of my moral doubts I no longer felt it. I could cut off my beard and I could confront the world with barefaced stoical indifference. In the mainstream the current I went with sometimes was vanity. In this all-night cafe I was scraping the bottom, but I would resurface again, not to career towards the weir in a dream boat to be broken in the rapids. I would find the calm waters of the estuary, and linger until the tide went out. Then I could walk away as someone who had been nearly drowned.

Looking out the dirty window, I could see the dawn rise above Edenham, off Notting Hill market, said to be built for suicides. But, still, takers were below average for a high-rise in London. It was strange that, despite the smog and run-down estates, daybreak could be so light and airy, a pink glow to warm the cockles. I wandered off, forgetting to pay for my breakfast. And nobody noticed.

The white-haired Rasta with his cross was not in evidence ('You've stolen my pain. You've stolen my death'). My body and mind seemed at variance. Walking was easy but thoughts came hard.

Could my future be in the hands of a dipso surgeon?

TOUCHING BASE

Cassandra was waiting outside my office. After a moment's silence, our eyes met, and then looked elsewhere. Metaphors may or may not clear the head, but my murky career was clouding over again. Cassandra had news for me. I would have to apply for my own job. The new chairman, Ivor Bell-Smith, had noticed my appointment as 'head' was as a stopgap for two years, and complained that I had dropped the 'acting' in correspondence. Employment law required the post to be advertised and open to competition.

The appointments committee would be made up of twenty representatives, including two Eminents, chaired by a Great and Good. They would be booked for the whole afternoon. Cassandra said that the interview would be three hours long, as I was the only likely applicant. I wasn't so sure.

I asked her when it would happen. 'That will be up to you,' she said. I wasn't in a hurry. I had only applied for a job interview once before (my first with Dr Thrower Up), and I wasn't keen to submit myself to an inquisition in open competition. I also knew that, as I had enemies in high places, I would be obliged to canvass support, and my pride baulked at that. Moreover, the trajectory of my murky career raised questions that could only be answered amongst friends. I had made my way by opportunism and by being difficult to place. I avoided too close a scrutiny of my curriculum vitae. During troubled times with the Upper Echelons over my Bright Young Specialists, Mal Combes had offered to get me anointed a Consultant, but I refrained, saying I didn't want a trial by sherry. That was not the only reason. Thanks to Hall McCall, I could boast a fellowship, but it was only the first part. I had kept that fact quiet.

I thought of reverting to a 'Projects Person'. I was well-positioned to contract myself out. Not having encumbered myself with a mortgage or family, money was only a secondary consideration. It would be good for my moral being. I fancied harnessing the Underlings in a groundswell of collective action (as in Renoir's *Le Crime de M. Lange*). The functionaries and professionals would be swept up into a tidal wave, and the Established Order would have no choice but to ride the crest. All this was possible, I thought, but only in the best of all possible worlds. But Voltaire was making a Dr Pangloss of me. I had gone beyond Ordinary Madness, and I couldn't just do what I liked. I had to put a brave face on what was expected of me. I was no longer a free man.

LOGGING THE BOOK OF LIFE

I put a 'Closed for Cleaning' sign on the door, and only came in after office hours to collect my mail. I had letters from Stanley O. Kay and Dame Brenda, both saying the same thing. The Eminents' new-found interest in quality standards was uniting them, but not sufficiently to jointly sign an agreed letter. They wanted to discuss the position paper on quality standards, which was to go to the Health Authority.

Dame Brenda suggested we meet in Lyon's tea house at Marble Arch. All the waitresses were near retirement age, and it was soon to close down. Dame Brenda ordered a cream tea for two and got down to business:

'The group thinks that Murdock ought to do the presentation. He had familiarised himself with Dean Slowey's clinical audit dossier, had spent time on the Reimbursement Board with Edna's index, and as a member of the Eminents, would be best placed to lead with my Delphic experts. If you step aside it would give your work the authority of coming from within. As you no doubt know, Murdock Gow is their one and only advisor now.'

Accidentally-by-mistake, Max Madison bumped into me a few days later, and the silver lining to my acquiescence was his rather gushy greeting. 'We are all impressed at your constructiveness, and indeed the group are thinking of putting you forward for a health service award for initiating a possible national initiative.' His bonhomie sat uneasily with his sarcastic self. It was mutually embarrassing. 'You must come to dinner with us sometime.' Eyeing the secretaries coming back from lunch, he remarked, 'Skirts are not only getting shorter but tighter.'

Schopenhauer was wrong. I wasn't going to be a fleeting catalyst. I was supposed to act as an agent in my own absorption into the Established Order. By effacing myself, all traces of their loose cannon had been buried. I was a far cry from my father's ersatz enemy, Voltaire, who started out in the law as an assistant notary. It wasn't until his writings made him a virtual outlaw that the emperors and empresses of Europe were lining up to dine with him. But Dame Brenda wasn't destined to be my Catherine the Great.

'Let the slime find their own cesspool,' I said, and went to the Bunch of Grapes, and got drunk. A rare event. I wasn't on my own (London Irish had won). Turlough McGee, the dodgy insurance man, put me in a taxi home. I feared I had signed myself up for Life or Death, but I had only bought tickets to travel to Dublin for a rugby international. Whether they were bogus or not I will never know. The trip was cancelled because of snow at Luton Airport. I didn't get my money back, McGee said, because I wasn't insured.

By the time I had slept off the hangover it was Monday morning. Masterful inaction would be my byword at work, I decided ruefully. I'd be nice to everybody, but respond to queries passively ('I need to think about it'). To pass the time, I logged everything that came my way in a personal Moby Book. It would be the basis of my job description.

I counted phone calls in and out, marking them for pointfulness; detailed the range of interaction with the Established Order; arranged memos into those that needed to be read and responded to, and those that should have been dealt with by someone else. I triaged complaints into warranted or not, or needing further investigation, and classified appointments in my diary into essential or a waste of time, and cancelled them all.

In sum, I sifted the necessary from the nuisances; shoring surprises against the expected (there were few) and, using weighted numbers, I drafted flow charts to identify positives, neutrals, and negatives and also drew graphs to denote progress or regression. It was a full-time job emptying my in tray.

Although curious about the consequences of doing nothing, the form of my loggings interested me more than the content. I wanted to keep the job description objective, and numbers and visuals served that purpose. But words, no matter how prescribed the terminology is, carry a degree of subjective judgement. As they flowed, my Moby Book not only recorded the job in hand, but began to analyse how it should be done. I was soon ranting self-righteously. The talking in my head had returned.

In adjudging the job, I was dramatising what Dame Brenda would call its 'agenda'. And she could also say I was 'dually accountable', doubling as protagonist and narrator. Egotism didn't come into it. It was Solomon's baby and couldn't survive sagittal sectioning. The self was subservient to the plot. The job was dramatising itself. Not me. I was only judging others as a footnote (to be deleted).

The talking shook its head and said, 'You are getting personal. As you did from the start with the job. Knowing nothing about management, you fell back on your experience of dealing with a world that you were not at ease with, that is, your childhood campaign to make your crimes and your mother's punishment commensurate. Whether to expiate the sin of being born, or your kinship with the prince of darkness, Mal Combes, you took a baiting stance. All the better to get a reaction in which your responsibles felt justified, but which served your purpose. They could let themselves go, and the release meant mutual catharsis so you were able to begin again and get things done together. You could get away with bad behaviour because after all you had the power. In short, you had recreated the job in your own image and likeness.'

I responded that putting a job in the place of my long-suffering mother made for a false echo. My boyhood 'run-ins' were willed. I conjured up reasons to justify her anger at the perceived 'errors of my ways', thus sinning by intention. Whereas, from the outset with this job, I was like a 'streetwalker in a town without pavements' (E. M. Cioran). My mistakes were not committed in full knowledge and therefore did not qualify as sins. It was the job that was in the wrong.

'Yes,' said the talking in my head, 'blame the job to morally justify your failure as a human being.'

I sighed and resumed my loggings. When the curtain finally comes down on my drama, I wrote, it will be impossible to say whether the play was a tragedy or a comedy. Virchow's ideas were my higher court, but it was one without jurisdiction. The real power was elsewhere. It could stop or delay what should happen at will, and then change its mind. Expediency was the law. My conscience was redundant. What would happen, or not, would be out of my hands. I was not so much a whipping boy as a whipping top. For me it wasn't a matter of 'getting away with it' any more, other than in thought. I had no reason for embarrassment.

The world had caught up with me and imposed itself, snuffing out the puffed-up ideas. They had nowhere to go except to run amok, or stay put like the proverbial mongoose before the snake, hoping to hypnotise it. The Established Order saw me as a prop in its stately pageant. I wouldn't have any lines. The best I could hope for was to be a spear carrier in the background. My presence would prop up their importance centre stage.

MURDOCK GOW

Cassandra asked me about the job description. 'A season in hell,' I floated, 'more Dante than Rimbaud.' She gave me a strange look.

I had reason for embarrassment. She let me know that Murdock Gow had made enquiries about the post. 'I am flattered,' I said, 'as it makes my job seem desirable.' It would be just another hat for him. Apart from his private practice in Harley Street, Murdock Gow had been seconded from the teaching hospital to my Bright Young Specialists' training initiative. He would need a deputy to cover for him when soaring elsewhere.

Mal Combes had dubbed Murdock, 'A clever young man, and no fool. He is going places.' I could see them dining together in the Gay Hussar. I found him agreeable, and working with him would be the best I could do if the worst came to the worst and he was appointed. It was very possible. I was over fifty and nobody could want my gay abandon any more.

I would have time to rein in my loggings and write articles on Virchow for philosophic journals. Foucault had brought medicine into vogue with his *Birth of the Clinic*. Virchow wasn't dead and buried. His law had never been given a chance to live. Its practical application had proved unrealistic in the present climate. But world historical ideas like his could stand up not only in print. Statues are built to them eventually. Maybe in a future era an enlightened politician will say, 'Sod-it! The world has gone to pigs and whistles. Generals, poets, businessmen, ayatollahs and automatons have failed as legislators. Only the banks and arms industry prosper. Let's all become doctors. Let the domain of medicine reign.'

The thought pleased me. I was indeed my mother's son. I was capable of what she called the eighth virtue. I knew how to change my mind. But I changed it again on second thoughts. And settled down to bumping along the bottom of my duties. My refrain, 'I'll think about it', chimed with my new resolve.

Michelle, who never complained, took me to task for unanswered letters and phone calls not returned, saying, 'I'm embarrassed making excuses.' People stopped trying to get through to me.

ASKING TO SEE BOBBY

At an Eminents' meeting, the group were embarrassed by my benign, disengaged air. Not only Murdock Gow, who had reason to be. Afterwards, Stanley O. Kay took me aside and asked me what was wrong. I expressed astonishment. 'Wrong? What wrong? I am perfectly happy with how things are.' An item on Lovecraft had been minuted. He had been removed from the Medical Register for two years. Murdock Gow said, 'Off the record, Reg Lovecraft effectively deregistered himself.' Pressed for more details, Murdock related how Lovecraft presented himself at the desk of the Medical Council, and asked to see Bobby. Now nobody except close friends call Robert Arnold 'Bobby'. So he was allowed into Robert Arnold's office. He was totally pissed, and begged to be struck off. Robert knew him by reputation and said, 'That's easy. We'll give you back the proportion of the subscription fee you won't need.'

Dame Brenda asked, 'Where is he now?'

'He's currently in a clinic in Turkey.'

Max Madison chortled to me, 'No Lovecraft. No payback necessary.'

Stanley was embarrassed. 'You don't have to worry, I will honour it.'

'What payback?' I asked.

'Angela told me she told you.'

'I thought she said, "Watch your back".'

'It's about Lisa Lemming's complaint against you. She comes from a highly respectable medical family. Her father is an old friend. We're getting her a job with the Reimbursement Board. You were right to note her clinical skills are wanting. Her forte lies elsewhere. Maths. Naturally she won't want to go to the tribunal.'

'So that's alright then,' I said, and he looked sheepish. At last I was disembarrassing my existential embarrassment by bringing it out in others, as Ian Russell had proposed. Hitherto I had found unburdening mine by, say, getting under the skin of staff who had reason to be embarrassed ended up with me being embarrassed on their behalf. Their leap from indifference to shamelessness did not include anything between. Now I had discovered that the best way to bring out embarrassment in others was to become an embarrassment oneself.

THE GOOD MAN'S DISTRESS

I started adding intimate footnotes to my loggings. It livened up the increasingly repetitive talking in my head. I kept the bottom margin of the Moby Book for doodling passing thoughts, or recording comments from friends like Ian and Joab. The latter was impressed by my withdrawal of industry and my chronicling of it. He faxed me Cordelia's invocation to tears on observing her father 'mad as the vex'ed sea', bedecked with 'idle weeds':

All blest secrets, all your unpublish'd virtues of the earth spring with my tears. Be aidant, and remediate in the good man's distress: seek, seek for him, lest his ungovern'd rage, dissolve the life that wants the means to lead it.

Maybe one day I would weep real tears. 'The good man's distress' was indeed a phrase used by Davy Crockett in his obituary of my father (I doubt if I told Joab that). Now I learned Shakespeare's words off by heart, and inscribed in my memory they were mine. But I noticed the next line in *King Lear* was, 'The British powers are marching hitherward'.

Still the secret scribblings were blest. My murky career had an achievable purpose again. Work was enriching my life by inflaming the imagination, giving me scenarios, rather than ideas. I had something to come home to, and my impatience to get back to my loggings was made even more piquant by putting off the moment. It was like my eldest sister who loved jelly, eating dry bread in between spoonfuls to prolong the pleasure. I savoured routine tasks of the day. They were not only part of the anticipation. I was pinning down my job with my pen.

I became more proactive in feeding the Moby Book. But I kept it to brief bouts of stirring things up. I wouldn't want to give the wrong impression to those who were embarrassed on my behalf. As my confidence in what I was doing waxed, my existential embarrassment waned to a sub-clinical level. I was at home with myself and others. At work and in my own time. In a small way.

Embarrassment returned me to my childhood. I was the red-faced boy furious with himself for betraying to his siblings through public jealousy his private yearning to be the cute Eglantine. It was a corrective, and reconciled me with being myself. On growing up, was it the saving grace that held me back from the brink of disaster and made sure I acted with decisive prudence? Or, was it the couch I put myself on, when ambiguity gripped me, to be my own shrink? As with all mind-doctoring, observing what's wrong does not mean you can do anything about it. Thus the glorying in what can't be helped.

Still I was in two minds about embarrassment. Did I need my ruling passion to save me from myself, or could it be a moral evasion, a luxury I allowed myself, to suspend judgement? Either/ or embarrassment wasn't merely social unease, and I feared that without it my ruling passion would be replaced by shame.

I worried also that by embarrassing others it could rebound on me by transference. In the small hours of the morning, when reading over my Moby Book, I felt sometimes that what I'd written was enough to embarrass readers. And I was one of them. I tore out a page and decided to test my embarrassment threshold by being petty. I gave a student on work experience a hard time after handing him a task, changing the instructions between inception and delivery. This was ignoble, I knew, since, eager-to-please, he dispatched the work immediately, delivering it by hand. The note I sent was delayed in the internal post. I ought to have been ashamed of myself. Instead, I said that if he had any wit he would have paused for thought before committing himself to paper.

The unfairness didn't cause me a morsel of embarrassment. My existential burden had been lifted to a higher sphere, or buried deeper in the earth. So pleased was I, that not only did I forgive the innocent party, but I praised him, saying he was an exemplar of Hegel's precept of hesitation, and his *sod-it, I'd-better-get-it-out-of-the-way* had avoided a Spurious Infinity. That is, paralysed by uncertainty, waiting, more in fear than hope, for fate to intervene… But as his grateful look glazed over I explained, thrilling to the thought, that on the horns of hesitation, by acting on the spur, he had found a point of application where anything was possible. I exulted on his behalf, although the talking in my head remarked, 'Bull.'

X

WEEDING THE GARDEN

'The love of justice in most men is simply fear of an injustice done to himself.'

—La Rochefoucauld, Maxim 78

ON THE THRESHOLD OF BAD BEHAVIOUR

I FOUND THAT RIDING A BIKE WAS THE BEST PLACE TO BE when I was in the grip of this state of exultation. The observer and the observed took a sporting interest in one another but were not emotionally connected. As I pedalled my hybrid at a steady cadence, I was rotating like the Earth. Riding the bike between meetings, the Grand Union Canal was my straight and narrow path to virtue. Along the banks of the canal there were the usual low-achieving anglers with their beer and Radio 1, and the odd loving couple wrapped up in one another. I had the towpath effectively to myself. I waved to the barge people passing by with their potted plants and yapping dogs. I was wheels with wings, listening to Schubert's *Winterreise* on my Walkman:

The nights are growing longer
and I'm going nowhere. Sleep
is a stranger I met once
upon a time. I was young
and curious. Now I've seen
it all, I cease to wonder
if I really belong here.

In my heightened state my mad, staring eyes were goggles and my twitching facial muscles a protective mask. My brainpan was a combat helmet, which showed my ears. A knight in cyclist armour is solipsism on wheels. But I didn't care what others might think. The excitement of moving from a bad state to an uncertain one had made me reckless. On or off the saddle, simmering traits in my character boiled over, and I became impatient with anyone who wasn't me. How could I possibly be subjective to them? I reverted to the deliberate rudeness I used to deploy with recalcitrant peer review groups. My beautiful temperament suffered the fool in me gladly. If I was heading for a fall, so what? I was enjoying the downward plunge.

I appeared at meetings with staff in cycling gear: lycra seeping sweat, luminous bike clips on my ankles and Bell helmet under my arm. Once I carried my hybrid into the boardroom and plonked it upside down beside me and gave its underpinnings more attention than what was being said. Cellular phones were just coming in and I was presented with one by a touting company, but I threw it out the window. I did not wish to be contactable at any time of the day by anyone. But as I spent more and more time sight-unseen in places where I could be myself alone, I acquired an old hospital pager and gave the number to my Michelle and nobody else. At boring meetings she paged me at hourly intervals. The pip-pip was a wake-up call, and offered an escape.

The pip-pip was sufficient for staff to assume it was an emergency or a call from above. I left without an excuse. If I was getting nowhere with them, I made a parting remark at the door. An extreme version would be something like, 'Sorry. I really don't have time for this. Work it out among yourselves and bring me something properly thought through tomorrow. Be sure it's in writing, because I don't intend on talking about it again. I'll make the necessary changes myself.' Then I sloped off, wallowing in their embarrassment, and my lack of it.

My stun-gun conclusion rendered colleagues into waxworks; pale, immobile, unable to speak or do anything. I learnt then how hate can't melt people down if they stay out of the kitchen, and say nothing. The next day what appeared on my desk was usually close enough to what I wanted, and I could be nice to everybody again. Although being by now shameless, I did not subject myself to apologising any more.

At meetings with the Eminents, I sported the cyclist gear more apologetically, explaining that a lack of time and facilities didn't allow me to change. I applied a Mennen stick to my wrist and neck, a strictly non-alcoholic deodorant. They were willing to be amused by my brazen flouting of the rules of costume, relieved no doubt that I didn't stink of sweat. The Mennen stick had the fragrance of a private swimming pool, I thought, and lingered in the air quite pleasantly. A clean smell.

Having to sit down is something I find difficult at the best of times. Working standing up like Hemingway is, alas, limited to pubs. And listening to a Dame Brenda Tabby or a Max Madison droning on *because that's what they do* is my idea of Dante's *Inferno* without the poetry. I had to balance the mood of a meeting against my tolerance threshold before deciding whether to stay or slope off (excusing myself with pathetic little Peter Lorre asides). The pager defence was less easy to get away with. But I flinched only when I sensed the prevailing tension would raise the offence to comment point. I switched the pager sound off and read the time. They could see the light flashing. Once I asked a question and didn't wait to hear out the answer, disappearing off wearing my 'Big Mig' goggles and Iron Man mask. Stanley looked shocked, and Max Madison laughed.

THE BENGALI OFFENCE

The pager defence was not my only method of warding off interruptions to my solipsist kingdom. I had the Bengali Offence for corridor and car park encounters: cutting someone off who, say, presented me with a report that I would have to rewrite for literary and/or ideological reasons. After whiplashing them with my tongue, I decamped, having delivered an ultimatum. There were no witnesses to such skirmishes. Harassment could not be invoked.

Usually my cut-throat interventions happened too fast for an on-the-spot reaction. Once an ex-army doctor was quick enough to intercept my exit by a fire escape. His bark ('How dare you!') brought the bite out in me. I put my finger on his tie and in a stevedore's whisper said, 'If you don't have that paper on my desk by Monday you're in it deep... Neither of us want that, do we?'

In the absence of embarrassment I was mugging up new thrills. Cheap ones, perhaps, but why walk the high wire without a safety net on the basis of a foregone conclusion? I was Rhett Butler in *Gone with the Wind* – 'Frankly, my dear, I don't give a damn.' The glint of playfulness in Clark Gable's eye depended on surprise. My actions were premeditated: a brutal bash and a quick getaway. 'The perfect crime takes no time,' I said to myself. But when I looked back I saw retaliation biding its time. Nobody could get away with behaviour like that forever. I didn't expect a dark alley, the whites of eyes and a knife in my back. But he who lives by the Bengali cut-throat…

Disembarrassed, my energies were more focused. I didn't change my mind with second thoughts. Things on the ground were getting done, but more out of fear than duty.

'Strategic bullying,' said Cassandra. 'It's unworthy of you.'

'Putting pressure on others to make what's supposed to happen happen is normal everyday management,' I said.

'It's a matter of degree.'

'If you said "kind" I'd be more inclined to listen.'

'That's Jesuit sophistry.'

'Skirmishing, used sparingly and without pleasure, has its place with self-satisfied Lollards.'

'But for well-meaning staff it's counterproductive.'

'Camus said, "I know what the soul of the well-meaning fellow is like, and it makes me shudder."'

'You needed to empower them, rather than yourself.'

'That's the received wisdom. Mine is that "democratic power is the long breath it takes to bring about change collectively. If, as the wind runs out, gentle persuasion isn't working, exercising coercion is sadly necessary."'

'Hmm. Sounds familiar.'

'Mussolini.'

'You'll end up in a disciplinary hearing.'

But at heart I knew that something was wrong. I was using power no longer out of righteous anger born of Virchow idealism, but for its own sake. It was becoming my plaything. In most sports management there are two types of petty tyrants. There's the trainer who knocks initiative out of his players. They defend well but lack the inspiration to score and the best the team can hope for is a nil-nil draw. Then there is the referee, who interferes with the free-flow by over-interpreting the rules. He kills the game. In either case it's boring and boredom is perverse. Troublemakers in the terraces run riot. For me management was a game of two halves, the first as an untrusting trainer, the second as a finicky ref.

My ungovern'd rage went too far with an inexperienced nurse on a home visit who stayed the night with an old man who begged her to. I suspended her for going beyond her duty, and being gullible. Ordinary loneliness is for the social services to deal with, I said. She was reinstated almost immediately by the intervention of one of the Great and Good. The press got wind of my actions, and threatened to publish her story. I was spoken to by Chairman Ivor Bell-Smith, whose wife worked for the Samaritans. 'Your over-zealousness showed the same lack of judgement as the young nurse.'

Chastised, if not chastened, I set up a workshop to devise a protocol for home visits. Details such as dress sense and whether to fix domestic appliances, or not, were hotly debated. I was particularly keen on replacing batteries in dysfunctional doorbells. A mischievous person leaked the draft to the *Nursing Gazette*, and it started a polemic about what nurses were for. Foolishly I wrote a letter to the editor, saying the best medicine is human warmth. The idea was much mocked.

But I was damned if the diminutive chairman of the board was going to take me to task for being out of order. In a follow-up letter I quoted without acknowledgement Diogenes, Descartes, Nietzsche and Foucault in defending my contention that it's the little things that matter. When Bell-Smith called me in again, and on the tips of his toes told me I was sabotaging the service by undermining morale, I couldn't help laughing in his face. It was a costly laugh.

HE WHO FUNCTIONS

Liberated from embarrassment, I saw myself as part of a cavalry, hoofed with logic, against an endemic enemy. My crusade had a theology behind it – the medicalisation of politics – but my working premise was that the big idea is the sum total of the little ones. Accumulation of what could be worked out, rather than attrition towards what couldn't, was the way forward in serving the god of common sense and humanity. In a small way, of course; being less a Don Quixote than a Sancho Panza, I rode a mule.

Still, I had my windmills. Mindful of Brecht's remark on Lenin ('He was a functionary, who functioned'), I thrilled to the thought that by functioning I might be a precursor of a revolution. The Russian revolution was started by a few hundred cells whose members were mainly clerks and teachers and had difficulty in finding time for meetings. But I perished the thought.

The idea was too big for its boots. My revolution would have to be a paper one. The articles for the philosophic journals would be manifestos on behalf of the god of humanity and common sense. However my former mission statement, 'Putting proven solutions into practice', would be moderated by substituting 'reasonable' for 'proven'. My working premise lacked scientific confirmation. Preliminary studies are never strictly proven, but they can be a reasonable basis for acting on.

As in the history of bureaucracy an incremental approach has an honourable place, and rationalisation, since the Age of Reason, has been a word associated with real change; science advances step by reasonable step. Agassiz in the mid-nineteenth century set the gold standard of research validation, and the bar is so high that it would exclude most of the recognised breakthroughs from being considered evidence-based. The post-Agassizian reputations of the two great biologists that emerged from the French Revolution, Geoffroy Hilaire and Georges Cuvier, exemplify the rise and fall of his negative hypothesis. Hilaire, who trusted his instincts, was regarded by scientists as a loopy theorist and Cuvier, who left no stone unturned, as one of their own. They were not wrong. Georges did the donkeywork, Geoffroy sucked his pipe and talked the talk. But recent research, most particularly the Human Genome Project, has reversed their reputations again, favouring Hilaire's hunches over Cuvier's honest endeavour. 'Accentuating the positive' is on the way back. Nevertheless, it's 'the mister in-between' that must broker the 'negative' and 'affirmative' for practical application *in vivo*.

It wasn't purely for historical reasons I changed my mission statement to 'Putting *reasonable* solutions into practice'. 'The proven', I knew, was the province of the Eminents. They fancied themselves as the keepers of the tried and tested. And respecting that would be a first step towards an *entente cordiale*. However, their predominant passion was keeping professional power in the political world proof from dilution. Common ground could be found in that as a baseline for launching Virchow. But somehow I couldn't imagine Max or Stanley on the barricades with me in a medical uprising, chanting a Virchow version of Al Smith's rabble-rouser: 'Yes, I have the proof that my city government is the sort of city government that the people of my city want. I could ride on a laundry ticket and beat those bullock-headed punks to pulp.' The Catholic governor of New York state in the 1920s liked a drink, and, despite Prohibition, at public meetings raised his glass of Wild Turkey to 'Your health, America'. He was loved, but lost the presidential election in 1928 to the 'dry' crusaders.

The Eminents were not much loved. In their new Established Order vein they were on the 'dry' side of progress which is 'ethical', according to Bertrand Russell, 'and therefore always controversial'. Maybe I could reconcile them to a more populist view. The small changes I had in mind were, I liked to think, obvious. The inevitable could be achieved quickly. It would be in keeping with my family's heraldic motto, *Fulminis Instar* (Like Lightning), and indeed Al Smith's governance. But I wondered would it bring them and me love, for what it's worth? And, if so, would it be our mutual downfall... Still, enough of windmills. The reality was more down to earth. I needed to be seen by the Eminents as more reasonable and practical...

I caused havoc with services to schools by banning leave-taking during term. This was particularly a problem for doctors with second homes abroad. I offered them the alternative of reducing their hours. Ground Forces revolted and I had my hands full avoiding a general strike. But those who bore the burden of having to increase their workload due to absent colleagues during the school holidays took my side. The doctors' union proposed employing locums. Service managers objected. Apart from the cost, it would mean more work, and you never knew what might turn up. And so it went round and round. In the end, I said, sod-it.

Dr Agata Brun confronted me, broadening the issue. 'I'm off to Tuscany for the Jewish holidays.' I countered her provocation, 'This sadly is a Christian country according to employment law. If you go you'll be hearing from Human Resources.' She became my designated enemy, fomenting trouble, a leader of her tribe. Freedom of movement, thought and religion were the battle cries (and anti-Semitism whispered). I compromised by offering Jewish holidays off if she was on call during bank holidays. I don't think it was ever taken up (she wasn't religious). The Muslim contingent observed all this with interest. Murmurs were that during Ramadan their hours ought to be reduced due to fasting and consequent fatigue. But observing that the Jewish lobby had got nowhere, they decided to be good.

I consulted Ian Russell on the Jewish dimension, and he said I had a persecution complex. But I knew I had to watch myself with Dr Agata Brun. And once again Chairman Bell-Smith called me in. She had been to see him. He suggested that since religion was becoming an issue, it should be subject to peer review. I said I'd talk to the Eminents, knowing they would not recommend any action. But I couldn't help being chuffed that my second step in the Virchow crusade, group audit, was his solution.

When Dr Agata Brun had a cancer scare, she was granted sick leave and passed the time in Tuscany. She returned part-time, taking work afternoons off to attend a clinic for 'prophylactic therapy'. I spoke to her: 'Attend in your own time, or your pay will be docked.'

'You can't do that,' she said. 'I'm a cancer patient.'

Bell-Smith took me to task. 'Your handling of this delicate matter is disgraceful.'

I stood my ground. 'My authority to get things done in a reasonable manner is being challenged.'

But Human Resources had been approached by another member of the Great and Good, and I relented. My functional working life was dissolving for want of the means to lead it. Passing Bell-Smith in the corridor, he warned me that the next time a complaint against me came his way, he would recommend disciplinary action. Voltaire had added a rider to Dr Pangloss's 'All is for the best in the best of all possible worlds': 'And the best is the enemy of the good.'

I experienced the good man's distress, and submitted to the vice of the virtuous: anger. But I tore up a letter of justification to Bell-Smith. Michelle nodded her approval as she binned it. I hadn't considered that being in the right isn't everything. Human considerations were above, and below, the letter of the law. I had stood my ground as a matter of principle, but I could not deny I didn't like Agata. And that could have contributed to my heavy-handedness over an administrative detail. Even the talking in my head had turned against me. 'When you do something on principle, and the principle is sound, but you have another reason, a personal one, that puts you in the wrong.'

'It's the story of human history,' I responded weakly. But my reasonableness was not that of others. I languished in what for me was a new sensation, the helplessness of not knowing what to think. It was to be tossed around on a hang-glider, not knowing where you were going to land. Voltaire, having advised most of the monarchs of Europe, concluded in the end that one should take strength from weakness. And so he wrote *Candide*. I searched out my copy, opened it at random and lit on: 'That's true enough,' said Candide, 'but we must go and work in the garden.' I went out and began weeding mine.

Starting with the dandelions. Their roots are the toughest.

DUMB-FOCUS

Block-head of services or simply a head-case, I didn't talk to people for three months. I spoke *at* them. My 'hello' sounded like 'goodbye'. I gave instructions and didn't wait for questions. If someone tried to buttonhole me, I waved them off with a 'not now'. I learned to scribble down what I wanted and hand the note to a courier.

My refusal was systematic. I counted the number of words I spoke every day. The ideal target would be fourteen, a word sonnet. My preoccupation with linguistic logistics wasn't a dodo race, but a serious game with a result. In cases when verbal communication was unavoidable, the ratio of my words to my interlocutor's was the score. The best result was when after a long speech I conceded a curt, 'We'll see'.

I answered questions 'yes' or 'no'. Never a 'perhaps'. I had learned from the One Ball Gang in college that that courts discussion. More dumb than deaf, I wasn't blind, cherishing the looks I got. The more puzzled the better. But my smiles and shrugs were eloquent. I used them to disarm, and distance intruders. At the Eminent Persons Group my near silence was not always taken as due respect, but, when tempted to make a remark, René Char's 'Silence seduces' came in handy.

I had become the inverse of the former 'verbal floater', and this stunned others' speech melodies. If I talked at all I echoed what they considered common sense. They didn't know what to say. At meetings I sat facing the door controlling the room with my eyes. A gunman entering would be in my sights. Nobody could get me. This was only half a joke. I felt uncomfortable, more in my body than in mind, and wished I was invisible.

'The body is an instrument, the mind its function, the witness and reward of its operation' (Santayana). I took an interest in nervous twitches. Compulsive chewers of biro heads, nail biters, neck and groin scratchers, ham-shifters, head-nodders, nose-pickers, players with little balls of paper, or bread pellets. And, above all, the leg shakers. What would have irritated me before touched my funny bone.

Stanley was a slumper. Max Madison picked his teeth. Dame Brenda crossed and uncrossed her legs, and sometimes tapped her feet. One of the younger members picked flecks (of dandruff?) out of his eye with a hanky. It impressed me that even Eminents had bad habits and forgot they weren't at home. Only Murdock Gow appeared relaxed. But to my shame I found the sharing of body space more interesting than sharing their ideas.

The twitchiness reassured me that the Eminents wouldn't be sitting there forever. Eventually, they would be obliged to stand up and stretch their limbs, or refresh themselves in the toilet, leaving me to lean back my chair on one leg, and drag it along the floor. The grating sound spoke to my condition. I had become a creaking link in the human chain that rattles along to no great purpose. In my dumb-focus, the talking in my head was a silent partner.

Things continued to get done. I kept a blinkered eye on what was going on, and made little changes as required. Every month since my days of Ordinary Madness I had scanned a handful of professional journals to keep up with the literature. I could almost do it with my eyes closed now. Poring over the abstracts was enough, and a quick glance at the graphs and tables of results. A Virchow-related subject would make me read an article. That happened about once a month. For instance, I came across a preliminary study on artificial hearts. I delved deep into the medical library off Baker Street. Mechanical hearts would take congenital weakness, and the confusion of personalities, out of transplants. But when it became evident that people would have to die to test it, I decided to wait until, as a solution to irreversible heart failure, it had living proof.

Still the prospect of *transhumanisme,* replacing organs with machines, had long-term prospects that would have thrilled Descartes: immortality by way of robotic body parts. However, its logical conclusion isn't life enhancing. Once the mind's function in mediating the body's performance is made redundant what else is left? Artificial intelligence boffins would be unlikely to fall back on the existence of the soul to make life worth living. They might be more prone to Schopenhauer's theory of the indestructibility of being, the immaterial will persisting after the body's death in an insentient state, waiting for a chance to be restored to an embryonic entity needing a mind of its own. But as secular scientists, depending on an evidence base, they would probably have to accept that, once functioning mechanically, the human vessel would merely be on life support, passing the time like a clock with infinitely rechargeable batteries.

Medicine is best left to Agassizian science. The negative hypothesis, like a chastity belt, can defend its virtue against the charlatans with messianic beliefs. The vaccine bugaboo was surging again. Stanley's emperor principle ('The ideal vaccine is one that everybody receives, except yourself') was being exploited by a surgeon I knew from my Ordinary Madness days. I had been studying unusual behaviour in a group of children diagnosed as autistic, accompanying them on visits to the dentist, the hairdresser, Lord's cricket and the National Gallery. I liked the routine and so did they. One of them made a cubist sketch of Bellini's *Madonna and Child*, and I showed it around after Roger Toussaint's Mortality and Morbidity Committee. The surgeon mocked my complicity with them, saying that I was probably autistic too. I decided to withdraw from the study as I didn't know what was normal.

Now the surgeon had surfaced in the media saying the mercury-based triple vaccine for measles, mumps and rubella was causing autism and bowel disease (shades of Dr Cotton). His evidence was based on a dozen children who had had the jab. Supported by autist action groups, and other lobbies including anti-fluoridationists, the tabloids went to town and the take-up rate for the vaccine dropped by half in London. Despite repeated research showing mercury was not a contaminant, measles and mumps would be back with a vengeance. It made me think that if Virchow came to power medical populism rather than science would take the lead. And my Hilairean approach, rather than being 'reasonable', would be sucked into it. The talking in my head remained mum.

The social historian R. H. Tawney's depressing conclusion in 1913 was no less true as the millennium approached: 'The continuance of social evils is not due to the fact that we do not know what is right, but to the fact that we prefer to continue doing what is wrong. Those who have the power to remove them do not have the will, and those who have the will, have not, as yet, the power.' Mrs Sibyl's Secretary of State for Education and Science said to a proposed renewal of Douglas's cohort study, 'I'll fund you if you tell me what I want to hear.'

I took to cycling in the graveyards of north London, a lizard in lycra wearing a black protective mask. In Kensal Green Cemetery I ate my sandwich on the empty grave of Sophia Peabody Hawthorne (d. 1871), wife of Nathaniel, the American novelist. The inscription stated, 'The Holy Sisters of Hawthorne, New York, founded by her daughter Rose (1902) to care for the dying, reburied the remains in Sleepy Hollow, Concord, with Nathaniel (d. 1864)'.

The cemetery catalogue said, 'We know from the one thousand five hundred letters she wrote to him that it was a great love story.' I didn't doubt it, but asked myself did they ever meet, other than to conceive little Rose? The inscription rather ambiguously read, 'Separated in death. Now reunited for all eternity.'

On my graveyard rides I rarely saw anyone. The dead have their visitors at the weekend. But on weekdays I had their company and the wildlife to myself. Butterflies and birds, and the occasional citified fox. They brought home to me that there was life after the death of my Virchow enterprise. I put the skeleton of a dead bird on Mrs Hawthorne's empty grave, and cycled down to the 'graveyard' of the Green Jackets, the rose garden in Regent's Park. Crossing the bridge I noticed it had been repainted. My final statement – 'Fire, water, air, stars, sky. Virchow lives' – had been erased.

HOSPITAL

'Put fresh events between yourself and your troubles. Break a bone.'

—Stendhal

The next January I was knocked off my bike by a white van on the North Circular Road in London. 'If there was traffic behind, you would have been a goner,' I was told on waking up in Accident and Emergency. 'Your right elbow joint is in pieces.' I was beginning to feel the pain. I made myself all small as I received an injection. Bouncer types in short-sleeved overalls rolled my trolley around and around corridors. The circles of hell came to mind.

I knew roughly what to expect from my days and nights with Roger Toussaint of Death and Disaster. Screws would be inserted to pin together the shattered joint, a technique developed in response to gun kickback injury during the Second World War. It is described as a council of perfection, which means it depends on experience and talent. If the operation failed, a metal elbow would replace the joint, and I would be effectively a one-armed cripple. Mr Hacker, the surgeon-on-call, was a recent arrival. We had been introduced at one of Roger's Mortality and Morbidity meetings. His dashing moustache and goatee recalled Douglas

Fairbanks in *The Mark of Zorro*, the silent movie. Apt, I thought, as he didn't speak. I had only his handshake to go by (off-hand was the operative word).

In a hypnotic haze I see a green pall of operation gowns about to envelop me. I'm stripped, my arms put in a white shift, and wheeled into the inner circle. The ceiling is fluorescent. Events are catching up with me. 'I'll have that,' a voice says. I see a forceps, a nurse's sky-blue eyes, a swab, a needle hanging from my arm, and a scalpel shining in the glove of a masked Zorro. As the sap of consciousness drains, the ceiling, lit up by a candelabrum, zooms towards me. I have just enough time to count the bulbs. Thirteen. I feel the first incision, a soft relief, and go under.

On waking, I saw from the theatre clock that I had been under for six hours. I wanted to shout, 'Give me back my life.' Not being dead, I thought better of it. As it was my first time under the knife, it never occurred to me that I would not consciously participate in the operation. My fearful sleep complex had been ambushed. I was not in touch with myself.

But I was playing blind-man's tapestry with what had happened to me. All I had to go on were loose threads. The strict routine of the theatre staff could be predicted, but it did not include being inside the patient's head during the operation, and so a repetition forward of the state of I was in would be at best a false memory. I had to think again. I was no longer at the cinema spiriting up the future to be lived. If only the brain had a 'black box' it would be possible to tell what happened to my mind in the interval between the dead sleep and the rude awakening. The engine of the brain is running at its lowest possible idle to keep the body alive. If it had an encounter with nothingness, as Mallarmé famously did in Tournon, I doubt it would have anything to report.

I had probably experienced nothing more than the 'sleep and forgetting', which Wordsworth oddly attributes to 'birth'. Did he believe our real life is in a pre-existence, and us coming into the world the Fall? In the womb, and before, our minds are too profoundly asleep even to have dreams to remember. But, sure as day follows night, we don't forget the reflexes that are preconditioned before birth in order to regulate our lives.

As my eyes accommodated to the light, the blur hovering around me clarified. 'I'm back,' I blurted as a smiling face came into focus. 'You were never away,' the nurse said. Her observation reinforced my feeling that the gap between what was and what is had narrowed to a point where I scarcely existed any more, and the present was a memory.

Waking from the void of non-being, and establishing continuity with what I was before, brought a rush of oxygen to the brain, and with it panic. My breathing quickened, and I flayed my arms around like a penguin in distress, loosening the straps that tied me to the bed. Assuming I was in pain, a doctor was called and morphine injected. A natural reaction had been suppressed by a chemical one. What I needed was a playback of the lost six hours.

On my second waking the nurses with their needles were replaced by the gloveless hands of auxiliaries. As the straps were unbuckled, despite my strong feelings on cross-infection control in hospitals, I appreciated the human touch. But I didn't feel free. I slid out of bed, and, listless, limp, my feet went from under me. I was picked up and fed some pills. But, still wanting to escape, I dissolved them in my mouth and spat them out with the water. The ruse revived my sense of having a mind of my own.

But, not being able to get out of bed, I didn't know what to do with myself. Was my body returning to me, or was I returning to it? Either way, it was a Cartesian impasse. So I said sod-it, and let the mind give way to the lower centres of the brain. The body began to obey the mind. It was a slow dance back into a life conditioned by reflexes it couldn't forget. The highlight was when I got up, crawled to the toilet and *walked* back.

I returned to life, going through the motions, eating and performing my ablutions, joking with the nurses, joshing with the auxiliaries. All my actions seemed like forward repetitions of memories from a former existence. And maybe they were. I wondered if I had misjudged Wordsworth. Maybe we are born to a sleep and forgetting, but as the brain grows we begin to wake reflexes that our antecedents evolved in blueprint. If so, the present contains the past and real time contains them both. Having reasoned thus, I fell asleep, forgetting the *Ode: Intimations of Immortality*.

On my third waking, I sat up and noticed that I was in an open ward. A vast space with a shanty of tents, beds enclosed by screens. I could only see one patient: a black boy whose screen had been moved to accommodate his extended family. I felt a twinge of envy and resentment. Here I was alone and abandoned in a public ward. But I was thinking more with my stomach than my head. Despite being fed soup and yoghurts at regular intervals, I was ravenously hungry. I saw the boy dig into chocolates. If I wasn't so weak I would have got up and gatecrashed his party. A sick man would not be refused a choice from the box.

My jealous greed moderated itself when I noticed the boy was on a drip. But if he could gobble down cream caramels there couldn't be anything seriously wrong with him. The rage of the famished welled up. If I could have committed a violence to spoil his feting I wouldn't have hesitated. But I was not near enough to throw a heavy object if I could find one. (Was there a chamber pot under my bed?) A spoon left behind after my last soup would merely cause confusion. I'd have to apologise, saying the missile had slipped out of my hand. I would have reason to be embarrassed.

My resentment turned to friends and colleagues. Nobody had missed me when I disappeared from circulation, maybe a day or two ago (I had lost my sense of time). They wouldn't have known where I was. But at the very least they could have phoned around the police stations and hospitals, and come rushing to my bedside bearing grapes and boxes of Black Magic. On reflection, though, I couldn't have faced visitors. My body had been insulted by surgery, and Job's comforters would only add to my humiliation. When the painkillers began to wane I was the one who would have to pretend that all was well.

When the nurse reappeared to take my blood pressure, she said I was normal. This was mutually gratifying, as though I had learned to behave, and was ready for exit management. The ideal patient is an automaton in the system, I thought. The quality of care is structural. The quality standards guidelines should make that its epigraph. I was thinking of work again for the first time in how many days? Nobody in this hospital where I had mixed my labour over the years had recognised me. I was absent on leave and, in my absence, performing credibly as a normal person.

I asked for a mirror. My face was the same as I remembered it. Left eye slightly smaller than the right. Uncombed hair and beard was to be expected. I licked my lips and pouted at myself, sticking out my tongue, and replicated the child-killer van Geloven's grimace, which resembled the one I cultivated when I wanted to frighten myself as a boy. But my face as an identikit photo of a serial killer was not how others saw me. When my name was mentioned, each had a look I gave them to remember me by. I perished the thought. Nobody but nobody would recognise the face of the minor monster contemplating attacking a boy on a drip. The nurse, seeing me smiling to myself, remarked, 'You must be getting better.' I threw her a van Geloven. 'Maybe not,' she sighed, and ambled off.

Mr Hacker appeared at my bed to discharge me. His three-piece suit was too imposing to give him an air of confidence. The moustache and goatee were gone and his chin was weak. He looked at my notes, but not me. Something more to add to the guidelines, I thought. I insisted on shaking hands. A metal shock went through my elbow joint. As his eyes were elsewhere he didn't notice the jolt of pain reflected in mine, and I couldn't resist remarking that it wasn't the first time we'd met. He looked at me, and out shot my official title, with a click of the heels, rather than a stand to attention. 'Yes,' I said, 'and I will be showing Mal Combes your handwork.' My mentor's reputation in the surgery world was such that my imagined Zorro swashbuckling on the battlements changed abruptly into the smug chap at the end of the TV-movie *Don't Make Me Angry*, who, having escaped from many perils, tees off on a golf course. On the third swing, he hits the ball which blows him up.

A less gratuitous ending than Godard's *Pierrot le Fou*, I thought. But Mr Hacker had every reason to be smug. His pins held firm. However it wasn't thanks to his aftercare that I recovered the use of the arm. I cancelled the follow-up appointment. I wanted to keep him in suspense. And I paid for it. For several months I had only one functioning arm. Until late one evening when my morale was at a low ebb, Joab and his latest girlfriend, an Australian physiotherapist, arrived at my house. Sylvia gifted me the necessary equipment for an exercise regime, and a form to apply for a sponsored cycle ride across Israel for the Mental Health Foundation. 'Get back on your bike,' she said. 'Tempting fate will be your salvation.'

After a few months the joint was functioning as before with two exceptions. I was no longer able to rotate my left arm enough to balance the hand on the handlebars of my hybrid to brake safely. So no more foolhardy mountain descents. And my little finger was dead. No matter, I thought. I have only played my violin once since my days of Ordinary Madness. Then I thought of my father. And felt pain.

CYCLING CRUSADE

Wearing elbow pads, I pedalled across the Holy Land, breaking with my left foot to mitigate the right hand's skid potential. Although it was springtime, and the almond trees blushed pink, the temperature by the Dead Sea was nearly forty centigrade, humidity ninety-five per cent. I insisted on wearing my Bell helmet, 'Big Mig' goggles and lizard lycra. It was a personal crusade. The 'I'm Not Mad' T-shirt was a wet rag. But, absorbed by the effort to keep going, it was a period of perfect blankness akin to what Nabokov recommends for peace of mind. Gingerly descending to Masada where the Gadarene swine went over the top, I arrived in Jericho, escorted by Palestinian police. I could hear the sonic boom of fighter jets overhead while being welcomed by children performing a fertility broom dance in traditional Arab robes.

We slept in kibbutzim, and under the stars in Bedouin tents. My fellow cyclists were 'All Human Life': doctors, nurses, church people, athletes, patients and their families. The mix was like an early 1960s movie: everyone playing up madly to stereotypes, but pulling together when the chips were down. I went along with it, but mounting the bumpy old road up to Jerusalem, and the steep climb to the Hebrew University, I got strangely competitive, forgetting it wasn't a race, and was the third rider drenched by a water cannon at the top. I knew then that I would be going back to work.

XI

THE NEW DISPENSATION

'Most terrible the bite of necessity.'

—Montaigne

THE CAVALRY

ON MY RETURN, AFTER ALMOST FOUR MONTHS, MY IN tray was empty. Michelle sang the praises of Murdock Gow who was acting-up for me. Evidently he had calmed down the Ground Forces. There was a corporate spirit abroad. People shared cars coming to work. It wasn't that he did much that would, or wouldn't, have happened anyway. It was a matter of style. Dr Agata Brun was a supporter. But still the bike parking that I had instigated was only used by him.

His handshake was hale and hearty. 'I've kept the coal fires burning.' He was keen to ask my opinion on so many things. Although officially my deputy, the general assumption was I would step aside when the post was advertised. I asked Murdock to continue as he did in my absence. 'I'm still far from myself. I've probably come back too soon.' Was I risking assassination like the bad boss who came back from the grave in Renoir's *Le*

Crime de M. Lange? The newspaper had prospered as a cooperative. The cartoonist shot the boss dead. Who would be my M. Lange? The list wasn't a blank sheet.

Cassandra told me that Bell-Smith was champing at the bit to advertise my post. I had a job description, but it was more like an apologia. I decided to revise it with Murdock in light of his experience. This would buy me time. He had reinstated formal meetings, but in lunch hours (with refreshments). He had style but where was the substance? Other than making himself available in a moderately refurbished office adjacent to the Eminents. His membership of the group was not challenged, conflict of interest, or not (seemingly the prerogative of the Attorney General applied to him. The top lawyer in the land could be a government advisor and minister at the same time). He asked for access to my files on peer review, though Dean Slowey had furnished him with copies. The title of his doctoral thesis was 'Criteria for Measuring Quality in Clinical Care'. It wasn't the counter-revolution. Murdock was everything I wasn't, but he understood my ideas, if not to the point of agreeing on Virchow (he thought it was 'too political').

I knew his amiable authority would make good staff better, and the not-so-good no worse. His task had been eased by the riddance of the dangerous clinicians. As quantitative targets were on the way out, low achievers would do less work. Arguably this would reduce mistreatments. Only a certain Dr Marcos worried him. The latest complaint against him was calling an Irish nurse a peasant. When she retorted 'Greek geek', the patients had to separate them. And it was the nurse that got the warning. I said, 'Leave Marcos to me.' I felt vaguely responsible for his evasion of the disciplinary net. Shades of Lovecraft, perhaps.

In my absence there had been a shock shake-up in the Established Order. The New Broom had been spurred into action by a spate of scandals: epidemics in long-stay hospitals due to dirty wards, and medical records disintegrating while extravagant computer systems failed (Roger Toussaint as always had anticipated the worst). Money would be found to restore health funding to its glory days. The New Broom had inherited Little John's belated economic boom.

Now that Mrs Sibyl had gone to her reward, mavericks like me, who feasted on the entrails of the Established Order which she exposed, had been overtaken. We were running on the spot waiting to be told what to do. Mal Combes was the exception. He had reconciled the Mandarins with the Eminents, and resumed his membership. As the young Eminents knew where their best interests lay, Stanley O. Kay's days were numbered. 'He always has his medical history book to go back to,' it was said. 'And his mother.'

The New Broom's analogies had given way to a new language, or rather a dead one warmed up. It derived from systems analysis brought in after the Second World War by American car manufacturers. It was all about managing the future, despite research showing that of the best laid plans drawn up by General Motors, and Chrysler, scarcely ten per cent were realised. The revitalised Established Order took to it. Maybe because they knew that.

The jargon had been around for some time in management training, and so fluency in it was rapidly acquired. Half-truths, like 'Patients First', were hailed as dogma (*pace* my father: 'the military wing of unreason'). Ideas were replaced by business wisdoms long past their sell-by date. A tidal wave of *mot d'ordres* from above flooded the working world, carrying all before it. The groundswell had the certitude of madness. Doubt was out.

It was as though Hegel's 'precept of hesitation' had been given free rein. Sod-it reigned supreme.

Catchphrases banish speculative thinking. Ideas are arias. Now that the hymn sheet was all recitatives and tinkling cymbals, vulgarities such as 'up for grabs' and 'on the money' vied with neologisms like 'value-added' or 'consumer-driven'. 'Cascading down' was not considered egalitarian, and was replaced by 'delivering outcomes downstream'. As was 'getting things done' by 'seeing things through'. But 'it must be seen to be' lingered on from the old Established Order.

However, the Mandarins still controlled by remote the purse strings, and hoops had to be gone through to get your hands on them. Cost-benefit hadn't been forgotten. Accountability wasn't just for accountants. Nevertheless the Mandarins appeared to be 'on message' with the New Broom. Having been silenced by Mrs Sibyl, they took to the jargon as to the manner born. They even had a code of conduct, a Nietzschean reversal – 'A servant to everyone and civil to the devil.'

MacCrone contacted me once to ask about the Bright Young Specialists and quality standards. His real reason was that a scandal was about to break. A general practitioner had been murdering patients. Edna Gray's analysis possibly had information that would indicate how long it had been going on. I had her early results from before the investigation was officially approved. After some hesitation I passed them on to him. Her prognostications, I gathered from Mal Combes, were supported by facts. But being unofficial, nobody in authority wanted to use the information in court.

It was not a good idea to question anything. The new dispensation gave merit bonuses to managers in exchange for freedom of expression. Whistleblowers became the terrorists of intellectual property. 'Speak to your line manager if you are unhappy. Resolve the matter internally,' was the watchword. The ultimate fear was that media exposure would damage the trust in the eyes of the New Brooms, and a public enquiry would be called.

Yet, at the same time, freedom of information was 'current money'. Fancy brochures with lots of coloured pictures were offered as annual reports. 'Transparency' required open disclosure of the balance sheet. But the rule of thumb could always be fiddled, as I knew well from Rami Bashir, the good sleeper.

Health Authority meetings used to be contentious affairs with lobbies in the audience baying for truth and justice (or Mrs Sibyl's blood). Not any more. Nobody turned up except loyal staff with aspirations, their relatives, and photographers. What appeared in the papers were the handouts. No more discord, dissent, devious dealings in the interest of 'seeing things through'. Everybody applauded themselves. Secrets – if not the truth – were out.

The surge of money should have excited the Virchow in me. Health was on the up (with motorway hard-edges and soft ecology). But politics hadn't changed, nor had the medical domain. They were still the professionally-led cabals that G. B. Shaw said were 'in conspiracy against the public' (though it was more with one another now). The New Broom's predominant motive, vote-catching, was a far cry from Nye Bevan's 'we ought to be proud... that we are able to do the most civilised thing in the world: put the welfare of sick people before any other consideration.' Whereas medicine now couldn't be further from a social science, when I started out health and social services were one and the same department. But they saw each other as competition for funding. A messy divorce ensued, and by the late eighties they were no longer talking to one another. When Mrs Sibyl announced, 'There is no such thing as society,' Voltaire's rider to Leibniz's *optimisme* was the last refuge of Virchow. It was possible her information was erroneous. The last hope was the same as the first: education. And where does that start? I missed Dean Slowey.

REDEMPTION BY DEFAULT

Since my accident I was consolidating: the main activity of iron bottoms. That meant doing nothing that couldn't be seen to be done. I had some experience of masterful inaction, but as the talking in my head remained a silent partner since my Israeli ride, I could concentrate on it without second thoughts. The word was my accident had led to a character change. Not for the worse, as would be expected. The shock, it was believed, had brought me to my senses. I had slowed down to the Established Order's stately pace. It made me a success in a small way. 'Our pet maverick has gone corporate,' said Dame Brenda. 'You could almost bring him anywhere.' True to say, I wasn't rocking the boat because I didn't want to fall out before landing on my desert island, retirement.

I submitted myself gracefully to a line manager. I accepted Consultant Connie Domebaste because she once told me that her husband thought he was Don Cherry. But being a paid-up member of the New Broom, she had moved up a rung in the Established Order, and we only met once. Her jargon was a stream of consciousness, and I was awarded a C-type performance bonus ('you could do better'). And so it was a relief to be facing the genial Pierre Rivas, the head of mental health. He didn't talk the talk, and his nods were as good as a wink. I expressed my doubts, that money wouldn't make any difference except increase the maintenance cost of new technology, and he sighed. 'Spending it is going to be a problem. Nobody knows where to begin.'

We got on well enough for him to confide that he had instructions to straight-jacket me into not giving Bell-Smith a reason to make trouble for the trust. I did not ask him where the instructions came from. I no longer cared. After that we spoke the same language, literally and metaphorically. His first language was French, and I was learning it, not merely to pass the time. And so our sessions became lessons. I learned the rudiments of *politesse*. He gave me a B-type bonus ('for good behaviour').

I confided my Virchow dream to him, and showed him the draft of an article I wanted to publish. I said I might even go on morning radio to talk about it. The opening made him wince. 'Medicine is the foremost science for the general welfare of mankind. And politics' prime function is to ensure the well-being of its citizens. Yet in this country the army is better funded, organised and respected by the government than the health service. The country is only at peace with itself when it's at war...'

'Go public with that,' he laughed, 'and say goodbye to your pension.' But I reassured him nobody would read it. Dick Cross had asked me for something for the Anarchist Society newsletter. He advised me that current policy on whistle-blowing was that it was unnecessary. It was simply a matter of reporting to the designated authority. I asked, 'Who could that be in my case?'

'Your line manager.'

'You, Pierre. I'm doing that.'

'I'll pass it on to my line manager, and so on...'

'Until it gets to the Public Prosecutor!'

'But, I suppose, the only proper authority is the truth,' he said wistfully.

'I'll pass that on to my line manager in hell.'

Pierre had worked in the same hospital that Jo Manders wrote about in 'Dentures in the Trees' and he too had suffered under the blimpish Dr Jebb. We talked about our days of Ordinary Madness. On hearing about Jack Black he seconded me to the Gang of Four set up to ensure HIV money was spent on it. Rami Bashir had shown that less than half of it was. Connie Domebaste was in the 'driving seat', which made me the passenger (the other two rarely turned up to meetings). But working with HIV specialists and patient advocates was quite different from anything I had previously experienced. Within a year two thirds of the budget had been 'ring-fenced' for HIV. And so, as a proven solution came with combination therapy, the money and expertise to put it into practice was 'in place'.

I found it easy not being difficult. And working to someone else's agenda was a change without progress, the iron bottom's ideal. Going nowhere is a comfortable place. You can stay there forever. People began to like me more. The Ground Forces were wary, but began to echo the Bright Young Specialists. Now sentimental about the Sibyl days, they were prone to say that without me they wouldn't have a job. Half true, but half a truth is better than none for a fragile ego. And my job felt more and more like 'a finite concern'. I was no longer essential. Now Michelle looked at me without alarm, kindly as one would an old retainer nobody had the heart to get rid of. My bathroom mirror showed a skinny veteran cyclist, hair and beard whitened, though eyebrows still black. Ageing, I thought, gives me the benefit of the doubt. But I hated the remark that I was 'mellowing'.

Pierre Rivas retired, and my new line manager was Tracy Harrow, an ex-Salvation Army general. The doxological conclusion to her opening sermon, 'What we need is a vision', made me look to the heavens. 'I mean,' Tracy Harrow said, not wanting to trade on her past, 'an idea.'

When Cassandra mentioned Bell-Smith was asking about my progress, I knew I would have to go sooner rather than later. I was fifty-six, and tired of being watched all the time in a Panopticon prison. At least I knew by whom. The European Court of Human Rights had found the gagging clause against whistle-blowers in breach of the law, and I entertained the notion of testing the ruling by writing subversive letters to the newspapers. I perished the thought, not wanting to give Bell-Smith the parting gift of disciplining me. Instead, once, on crossing him in the corridor, I fingered my brow, bowed deeply, murmured, 'Salaam Master,' and made to kiss his hand. It was my last deviation from the received norm, and nobody but he heard me. As a block-head of services, or a head-case, it was a less than heroic bid for freedom.

I managed to slip in a reference to Virchow in Murdock's doctoral thesis, and completed the article for the anarchists: 'Fire, Water, Air, Sky, Virchow lives.' I copied it to Nasty, and Mal Combes phoned me. 'I want you to do something for me, Poet. Go while the going is good. You're young enough to do something else. But for a change I want to do something for you. I think I can wangle you an honorary fellowship with the royal college. It will annoy everybody.' However, knowing my

CV wouldn't pass muster with them, I laughed it off. 'I've always been a mock turtle, and have no wish to be a real one. Now I'm retiring into my shell.' He promised not to try to tap me out.

The Health Authority accorded me a bonus: a back-payment for acting as a Consultant without being anointed one by the royal college. In effect, I was elevated to the Upper Echelons, retrospectively. Nothing in my murky career was ever the right way around. I was always somebody's Trojan Horse. This time I had nothing to hide in my belly save that I was slipping off with a fiscal kiss. I didn't reproach myself. The writing on the wall was clear: 'Your kingdom is to be divided. Share in the spoils, in a small way.'

During the handover period I disappeared from sight. I cycled down to the Victoria Embankment on the off-chance of spotting Madge Herron. I thought of Ireland and she came to mind. But, like the family home in Cork, she had disappeared. After my mother's funeral the house was sold. Michael told me it was to be knocked down to build a modern mansion. I never returned to haunt its renewed ruins. I didn't want to be my own ghost.

At my next Sunday whiskey with Ian, he showed me Madge's obituary in *The Guardian*, and I learned that she didn't end her days homeless. One of the young poets, no longer young, got her a place in a nursing home, but as an open patient where she lived the life of John Clare. In and out at will, shouting joyously in the streets, the streets that she loved.

I revisited Søren Kierkegaard. McFee's copy of *Either/Or* had saved me from a fate worse than the 'perhaps' of the One Ball Gang. And so in the last six months of my paid employment his writings absorbed all the functions of my soul. It was the *grand sinderesis* of a purgative, a scholastic sneeze that opened the philosophic portals so right and wrong and good and evil seemed clearer until you thought about it. Poor Søren had got himself into self-complicating impasses through trying to live an idea. When things did not work out as hoped – the life kept changing and so did the idea – he learned to live with the consequences by writing about them, until in quiet despair he found a pretext 'for stealing out of life' as though he had 'forgotten something'.

Work, like genius, is ninety-nine per cent perspiration and one per cent inspiration. For many years mine had been the other way round. But as the Madness became less Ordinary, the inspiration suffered and, folly by folly, it receded into the received wisdom of 'dogged does it'.

'Whatever the play, the last act is always bloody,' says Pascal. I'm not so sure. The comedy of my career didn't end with undue blood on the carpet. Pride tended to come *after* a fall, and I picked myself up to save myself further embarrassment, saying that I had an idea to get away with. Nobody need know.

However, I wasn't made for the long sweat to *point* Rolex. And so I would take myself off to find my inspiration elsewhere. I chose a less temperate clime, where if it doesn't come, I can always perspire, sitting snoozing in the sun, dreaming of a better world.

But I had one last thing to do before slipping away.

Having promised Murdock Gow to sort out Dr Marcos, the complaint-resistant misanthrope, I avoided the confrontation. Marcos was the incarnation of dead bat, and, as it was an aspect of myself I had managed to leave behind, I didn't want to meet a version of my former self on the way back, like in a film reel in playback. But I had to face my past, if only to face the future with a clean slate.

TEARS ARE FISH WITH LEGS

Dr Marcos's resemblance to Omar Sharif does not include the dewdrop eyes. The sockets look empty, like a Greek statue that has had its lapis lazuli plundered. Nor has he the romantic allure. A bachelor in his fifties, he shares with the star of *Oh Heavenly Dog* an unrequited passion for bridge. When cornered, I was warned, he plays his cards close to the chest, one move ahead. Nothing can touch him.

I wait for Dr Marcos to start his car, and tap on the window. As he rolls it down, I open the door and invite myself in. 'I want to talk to you.' So on a cold, wet, late Friday afternoon in November 2002, Dr Marcos and myself are sitting in his Volvo with the engine running, night falling on a washed-out Portobello Market, no sign of life, not even a rat rooting in the grain. I'm throwing him the line that early retirement would give him a chance to fulfil his potential at the card table.

I'm hoping to surprise Marcos into agreeing with me. But years of warnings without a disciplinary hearing have given him a righteous smirk. 'I'm invulnerable.' I flourish a fistful of letters. 'These are complaints from colleagues and patients. There are so many people unhappy with you, you must be unhappy yourself.' Marcos doesn't need to stiffen. The empty sockets see nothing, save his own reflection in the windscreen.

Our breath is fogging up the car. I remark softly, 'At our age there is surely more to life.' The smirk moderates into a patronising smile. He realises I'm not just talking about him. The wipers are like double slaps in the face. I can't find anything more to say, or do. It's enough to make one weep, I think. The thought recalls for me anew McMaster performing *Othello* to a rowdy audience in a Limerick cinema after the last showing. Instead of enacting the famous epileptic fit, he burst into tears. This silenced the hecklers. His concluding 'die upon a kiss' received rapturous applause.

I bunch up my features and, although I don't actually produce tears, or introduce sound effects, my snivel is convincing enough for Marcos. 'Please, please. You must control yourself. And be strong. We need you to be strong.' His 'we' takes me aback, and I feel a strange welling-up of affection towards the man I loathed a minute before. I'm moved by his concern that I'm needed for the good of more than myself. I let myself go, and he puts a hand on my heaving shoulder, saying, 'There, there.' I wasn't bluffing. After the initial blub it was a relief, and I sobbed, 'Medicine is a social science, and politics is nothing but medicine on a larger scale.'

I succeeded by default. My loss of pride restored his and, in his case, pride came not before a fall, but a change in position. The moment of subjectivity towards one another achieved a mutual objective. He went along with the early retirement plan like a soldier to a marching song. And so, in a washed-out market my working days ended on a soggy note...

A REPETITION
FORWARD ON MY WALL

As I write, on the wall before me I have two photographs taken in the late forties. My parents, Michael and me. The first is outside Woolworths on Patrick's Street. Behind us two men in felt hats and three-piece suits are standing together, talking at a commercial angle. Each has an umbrella. One of the umbrellas is open and the taller man is spinning it.

My parents and Michael face the camera. I'm turning around to look back. You can see it's a fine day because there are two young women in summer frocks cycling on the far side of the road. There are five parked cars, boxed Fords. A Dodge Deluxe is about to pass the bikes. The only background detail I recall is not in the picture – wedding guests coming out of the Victoria Hotel. The bride wore green taffeta. I'm holding the hand of my younger brother Michael, a pretty, forward-looking boy with curly hair and a buttoned-up white shirt. My trousers are from my first communion suit. The jacket has been replaced by a light pullover. My shirt collar is sticking out and the crooked tie looks as though I knotted it myself.

My father is fifty years of age; the great mane of whitening hair brushed back reveals his high forehead. He is not acknowledging the camera. The camera is acknowledging him. His indifference to it tempers high seriousness with humour; hands resolutely in his pockets, knowing he is every inch the thoughtful professor walking out with his young wife and two boys. Her arm brushes his elbow.

My mother is slender in a dark suit of the period, high shoulders and narrow waist. The white blouse has a cravat, and the summer hat is tilted so her dark hair, tied back, shows through. She looks directly at the camera, defying it, submitting to the intrusion with apparent good grace.

The second photo is on the Grand Parade across from Woodford Burns, the claret merchants. My parents are no longer side by side. Michael and I are between them. It must have been the same day, as the clothes have not changed. I'm facing the camera this time, like my mother. I don't quite match her alertness to its eye. But I'm doing my best. Michael appears sulky, as though he wanted to be next to her. My father is looking into his own thoughts, dissociated. He might almost be about to take off in another direction. My mother is swinging her right arm, relaxed enough to challenge the camera, confident in the knowledge that she has got her look right. My father's abstraction may be an awareness that he got it right the first time and that that should have been enough.

I like the first picture best. The family walking together to my father's mild satisfaction, my mother's determination, Michael's sure step, and I am looking back. For a moment we are the guests of the street photographer, and one another. Welcome enough, but laterally there are accommodations to be made. My mother is making them.

The camera has registered a repetition forward, renewing in my mind's eye a happy summer's day like any other sixty-five years ago. While what's in the background is in the past – a business deal, a wedding and the passing fair – we are ever present. And I, for one, am proud to be there.

THE ESTABLISHMENT PECKING ORDER

THE POWERS THAT BE

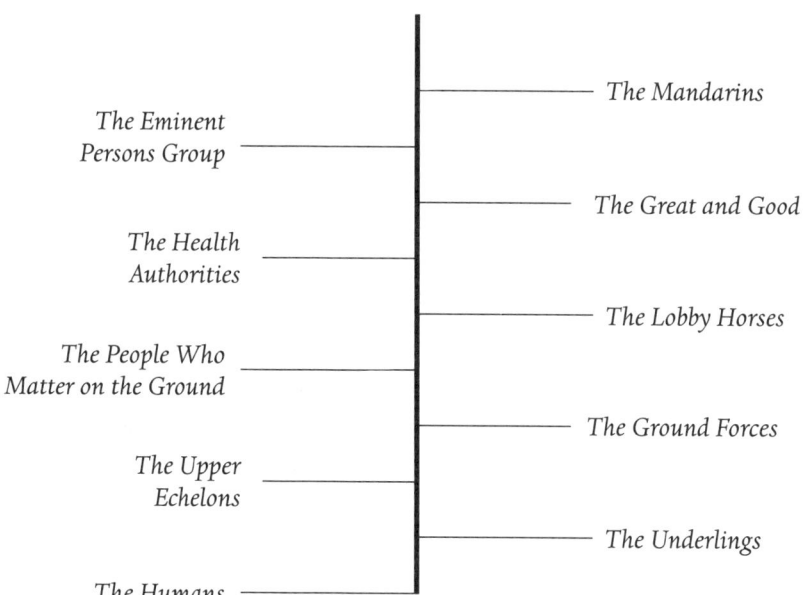

The Eminent
Persons Group

The Health
Authorities

The People Who
Matter on the Ground

The Upper
Echelons

The Humans

The Mandarins

The Great and Good

The Lobby Horses

The Ground Forces

The Underlings

both knew he had to do better than that. Heat ripped through Anne's body despite the icy temperature, and an eternity passed before Fleur looked up at them, a trembling mess of indecision.

Now James. It has to be now …

The athletic police officer warily descended the thin ladder, reaching out, beckoning Fleur to him with his free arm, his voice stronger this time.

'Hold on to me, Fleur. I'm going to take us away from all this.'

Better, much better …

There was a crunch. The sound of Fleur's foot slipping.

'Shit … shit … oh shit …' the young policeman panicked, grabbing out at flailing arms while keeping his left arm hooked firmly around the cold metal frame.

Unable to watch any longer, Anne banged her forehead repeatedly on the cold, unforgiving concrete. Her old behaviours returning, but withholding their promise of momentary ease.

Please Banksy, I know we did wrong, but we can fix it. There is always hope …

The sound of hoarse, otherworldly grunting filled the air as the young officer yanked Fleur towards him with all his might. The ladder creaked with the extra weight, and she dared to look down at his jutted chin, his sinewed neck of nubble and steel